Nancy Beckerman has written a[n] encounter with, and resolute response to, a formidable illness. A sad, moving and captivating book – I couldn't put it down…
—Michael Weissman, M.D., Physician

Nancy Beckerman shares a spiritual journey of fear and hope, a story of strength and beauty of the human spirit, in *Out of Time*. Nancy became, as she writes, "an example of how to deal with cancer," one we can look to in understanding the fear, optimism, honesty and love that comes with a family's fight against cancer. Having walked this path with the Beckermans, it is a story I will not forget; nor will those who experience it through these pages.
—Jonathan Lewis, M.D., Ph. D., ZIOPHARM Oncology
Formerly Professor of Medicine & Surgery at Memorial Sloan-Kettering Cancer Center

MUST READING for medical students and everyone else in the medical field and its support services, including those who work in the medical insurance industry, caregivers, and everyone who comes in contact with patients.
—Susan Milligan, Caregiver

Out of Time is an honest direct, moving portrait of a couple battling cancer together. This is a must-read for medical professionals who want to understand illness from the patient's point of view, and how a doctor can become a "guardian angel." It shows how possible it is to find moments of joy and repose amidst adversity, and how we can hold on to love and life even when facing an overwhelming loss.
—Ilana DeBare, Author of *Where Girls Come First: The Rise, Fall and Surprising Rise of Girls' Schools*

A life-affirming journey of two people facing cancer with love, courage, determination, humor, and, most of all, hope. Required reading for anyone navigating cancer treatment.
—NC Tenenbaum, Owner, MedicalFrontiers.com

If the story of the loss of a beloved husband and father could be uplifting and positive, then the author of *Out of Time* has made it so through her thoughtful and heartfelt telling of this very personal tale. Nancy Beckerman slowly peels back the layers of the story, taking the reader through a journey so many of us will go through, and gives us an important lesson on how to get out of a tragically early death of a spouse – alive and with hope for the future.

—Zazel Loven, Editor, Writer, Community Activist

With careful documentation, this well written memoir of a loving couple's struggle is very compelling reading. It was sad but always hopeful.

—Polly Wastcoat Weissman, Teacher

OUT OF TIME

One Couple's Journey Through Cancer

Nancy Greyson Beckerman

Out of Time: One Couple's Journey Through Cancer
by Nancy Greyson Beckerman

Signalman Publishing 2011
www.signalmanpublishing.com
email: info@signalmanpublishing.com
Kissimmee, Florida

Cover design by: Joel Ramnaraine.

Photograph on front cover by Barry Beckerman.

Author photograph on back cover by Whitney Lane Photography.

ISBN: 978-1-935991-19-9 (paperback)
      978-1-935991-20-5 (ebook)

Library of Congress Control Number: 2011938246

Printed in the United States of America

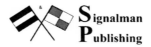

Dedication

This book is dedicated to Dr. Jon Lewis, our guardian angel; to the many medical people who showed us dedication and compassion; and to our family and friends who supported us with love throughout our journey.

Preface

This is my story, the story of an ordinary person facing extraordinary circumstances. It is a testimony to the strength which is inside all of us, which we don't know we have until we call on it. To the love and good will of human beings towards each other, which you don't think is there at all, but which surfaces when you need it. And, as our doctor once said, "to the human spirit."

Acknowledgments

I would like to thank my family and friends for their ongoing love and support. You made this enterprise possible; you were there when I needed you; you helped me heal. From the bottom of my heart I thank: my close friends, my swimming pals, my karate friends, my Sensei, my book group, my meditation teacher, my friends at CAN, my Sunday movie buddies, my school friends, my amazing cousins, aunts and uncles, and, lastly, my wonderful brother and his wife and family, and my miraculous daughters and son-in-law. How lucky I am.

Special thanks go to Phyllis Ross for her editorial expertise and her kindness.

PART I

THE ILLNESS AND THE BATTLE

Chapter One

Discovery
(May '98)

It's funny how one moment can change your life forever. One split second and nothing will ever be the same. Ever.

It was May. Seattle was beautiful. We were on vacation, enjoying Lake Washington and the Cascade Mountains, visiting our daughter Sara and her new husband Richard. We had hiked in the mountains, strolled by the falls at Snoqualmie, relaxed by the shore of the lake, and ridden the Washington State ferries. We had discovered a nature preserve in Kirkland, just outside Seattle, where we found eagles nesting, along with big turtles sunning on logs. With one more day left before flying home to New York, we had had dinner at the home of an old college friend of mine who lived in a nearby town, and as we drove back to our motel the wind was fierce and it was raining hard. The drive took about 45 minutes, and by the time we reached our destination, it was pouring. The roads were treacherous and the trip had been stressful, especially since the area was unfamiliar to us. We were happy to reach the comfort of the motel, and because it was late, got ready for bed.

"Nan, look at this!" My husband's voice demanded my attention. "Look at this." Three little words. The tone of his voice was chilling. I looked at his leg. There was a bump on Barry's inner thigh about the size of half an orange. Out of the blue. It was big. It was hard. My heart sank, and I froze. Whatever this was, it was terrifying. How had this happened? How could something like this appear so suddenly?

This was the moment of change; nothing would ever be the same again. We were not invulnerable. What had caused this huge lump to appear so suddenly in the leg of a normal, healthy, physically active man in the prime of his life?

Thoughts flooded my mind; what should we do? Book the next flight home? But it was Memorial Day weekend, and we probably couldn't reach our doctors anyway. If we stayed in Seattle for the last day of our vacation, we would get home as the holiday weekend ended, and could call our doctors immediately. Or should we call them right now? I tried to remain calm, knowing that we had an emergency on our hands.

Barry's voice broke through my thoughts, telling me that he thought he had pulled a muscle in his leg a week or so ago while swimming, which we did almost every day. He thought he remembered being too vigorous one morning, possibly injuring a muscle. It was hard to remember. Then again, the rental car we had been driving for the past week was extremely low, and every time he had gotten in and out, he had been straining his leg. Maybe he had injured his thigh or had torn a muscle, and perhaps it had bled, causing this mass to develop. He was using his medical training to try to explain this alarming development. In the end, we went to bed, fearing that we had made a terrible discovery, hoping that we were wrong.

We spent the next day with Sara and Richard, trying to enjoy our time with them, not to alarm them, but we were distracted and worried. We returned to New York on our scheduled flight, and the next day went to work at Barry's office and called our internist.

The doctor wanted to see my husband immediately; he knew that since Barry was a physician, he would only report a true emergency. At the lunchtime appointment, the doctor didn't know what to make of the mass. It was not typical of anything. He suggested an ultrasound, and after work, my husband went for that test. I was home when the phone call came: Barry's voice was weak. "Nan, could you pick me up at the x-ray department?" I jumped in my car and sped over to the medical building. My husband hadn't wanted to tell me on the phone, but the radiologist who had read the ultrasound thought the mass might be a tumor. It looked suspiciously like more than a blood clot. The next step would be an MRI the following morning at our local hospital. By this time, several days had elapsed since we had discovered the mass, and it seemed to be getting slightly smaller. We found this reassuring.

As we conferred with the young radiologist who read the MRI, we asked him whether a tumor could get smaller. He replied that it could not. Again, we sighed, grasping at straws. The radiologist, a friend and also a patient of my husband's, someone he often ate lunch with at the hospital, continued speaking, suggesting that we repeat the MRI in about a month, perhaps even get a consultation at Memorial Sloan-Kettering. "But it's getting smaller," we answered. Barry refused to consider Sloan-Kettering; he did not have cancer; at Sloan they would treat him for cancer, and he did not have cancer. And the mass was certainly getting smaller. Tumors did not get smaller. How many times did we tell ourselves that?

Over the next month or so, Barry examined his leg every day. The mass was indeed getting smaller, but almost imperceptibly. Every once in a while, we discussed possibilities. If this were a blood clot, it should be getting reabsorbed by now. If this were a tumor, it might be a sarcoma. If it were a sarcoma, he was a dead man, Barry said. This he had learned in his medical training: sarcoma meant death.

Finally, we decided to consult a local orthopedist. The doctor was very young, and the diploma on the wall told us he had graduated from the same medical school as my husband, only about 30 years later. He, too, was stumped. This lump was not typical of either a tumor or a blood clot. The doctor wanted us to wait a few weeks and then return to see if there was any change.

As the summer passed, a nagging fear lodged in the back of our minds. Unspoken was the suggestion that we go to the cancer hospital in the city. It became clear that Barry's leg was not getting better. Then the pain started; the orthopedist prescribed pain medication, which my husband took for a while.

Somehow, we found time and energy to get away for a week-end that summer. We drove to Ithaca in upstate New York, where we both had gone to college, and where we often spent weekend getaways. There was a lot we loved to do up there, both on and off the Cornell campus. We knew all the state parks in the area, and enjoyed the beach and marina on Cayuga Lake at Taughannack Park, and the many waterfalls at Enfield Park. The college bookstore could keep us busy for hours, and then there were all the walks up on the campus, around the gorges, and down in the old, historic town.

This time Barry's painful leg kept us from doing much walking. Even so, this mini-vacation took our minds off our worries a little.

Near the end of the summer, we were supposed to go to the city to see "Alice's Evidence," a play created and directed by our older daughter, Ellen. The play was part of the Fringe Festival, which was taking place at the Henry Street Settlement Theatre in lower Manhattan. We wanted very much to see the performance, and Ellen had asked Barry to videotape it for her. This experience was special for me, since my own grandfather had grown up in that neighborhood, and had spent time during his childhood at the old Henry Street Settlement building. What would he say if he knew that his great-granddaughter was directing a production at this very place?

We went to see the play, driving down to Manhattan; we parked, and then had to sit in the car while Barry rested his leg. We ate a picnic supper in the car, since he couldn't walk any distance to a restaurant, and even found it painful to sit in a chair. When Barry felt he could make it, we got out of the car with the video-camera, and made our way into the theatre. We were allowed in early to set up the camera. We certainly would not have been able to stand and wait in line. Luckily, the theatre had very soft, comfortable seats. I will never forget that evening: seared into my mind are my husband's pain as we sat there, trying in vain to concentrate on the vivid performances of the young and talented actors, our daughter's pride in her work, and, underneath, the deep concern we all harbored about my husband's condition. Attending Ellen's play was one of the last "normal" things we did that summer.

Back home, I wondered whether the lump was getting larger; *was it just my imagination?* At some point we became conscious that we were deluding ourselves, wasting time, denying, denying, denying. It had become painful for Barry to stand and walk, and still he was working in his office, seeing patients, even performing surgery, denying, denying. We had to act. The orthopedist ordered another MRI, and when the radiologist read it, the mass was clearly larger.

What we needed now was a specialist, but who? How do you find a specialist when you don't know what's wrong? In some ways, this week was the worst for us emotionally: not knowing where to turn, or whether we could even find the doctor we needed. It is awful to feel that something in your body is out of control, and you don't know who, if anyone, holds the key to stop it. The local orthopedist recommended another orthopedist in the city, and we made an appointment with him, but with misgivings. If this was a tumor, did we really want an orthopedist? My husband consulted another colleague who specialized in cancer, asking him whom he would recommend. He suggested a well-known surgeon at MSKCC (Memorial Sloan-Kettering Cancer Center), and was kind enough to call the office for us; we made another appointment. At this point, once we faced the inevitable, we couldn't wait to see the specialists, and to find someone who could handle the problem, and not say, like the others, that he had no idea what was going on. Meanwhile, Barry was in considerable pain daily.

CHAPTER TWO

MEMORIAL SLOAN-KETTERING
(Sept '98)

The appointment at Sloan-Kettering was late on a Thursday afternoon in September, and it was not with the well-known surgeon, since he was out of town. The appointment was with his associate, Dr. Lewis. As we sat in the waiting area, I looked around at the other patients and their families, all of them dealing with cancer. Some looked ill, pale, thin; some were holding canes or were in wheel chairs; some were bald. Yet some looked okay. We had entered another world, through the "looking glass." It was a world we hadn't wanted to be a part of. But who does?

Since the decision to seek help in the city, we had been numb, in a state of anxiety, super-vigilant. You know how people say fear is their constant companion? It's true. You wake up every morning, but the bad dream doesn't go away.

We sat in the waiting room for a long, long time. The doctors were working hard; they were overworked. I didn't mind waiting; I felt appreciative that they had squeezed us into their schedule at all. I was afraid of what the examination would reveal. We didn't know what to expect, and we still had our appointment with the orthopedic specialist at another hospital scheduled for the following morning. We wanted to be able to decide which doctor would handle the case after we had met and spoken with each.

A nurse came in and called out my husband's name, and we followed her down a corridor and into a small examining room. She asked us questions, and we relayed the history of the mass: its appearance, apparent decrease in size, and finally its growth and the pain it was producing. She was very kind, and it was comforting to be with someone who dealt with dire situations like this as a routine. Then we waited for Dr. Lewis, prepared for anything.

At last, a husky man with a baby face and dark, curly hair strode into the room, his lab coat flying behind him; he introduced himself, and shook hands with us. Dr. Lewis. My heart sank; he looked so young! How could we entrust Barry's life to anyone so young? We were desperate, and knew we had only one chance to choose a doctor, and our decision had to be right.

The doctor started speaking with a lilting accent; he exuded confidence. *Well, maybe.....* He examined Barry's leg, talking and asking questions all the while. I was taking notes furiously, knowing I wouldn't remember what I needed to if I didn't write it all down. My mind was a blur. Finally, Dr. Lewis said that he didn't think that it was sarcoma, but if it wasn't he would have to find out what it was. *Imagine! Someone taking charge, and saying that he could and would find out what this was!* He asked us if we could wait for a while, as he wanted to take my husband's scans out to consult with some radiologists in the building. Of course, we would wait! When he left the room, Barry and I looked at each other and knew that this was the man we needed. Little did we realize that he would turn out to be an angel in disguise.

While we waited, Barry and I wondered: dare we believe that this lump was not a sarcoma? We didn't want to get our hopes up, just to have them dashed. We waited and tried to imagine the radiologists examining the MRI's, and hardly knew what to hope for.

Eventually, Dr. Lewis returned with the news that the radiologists couldn't tell from the scans what the mass was. They recommended a biopsy, which Dr. Lewis could do right then and there, if we wanted. We nodded at each other; we knew we would do whatever this man suggested. Within half an hour, Dr. Lewis and his assistants had numbed my husband's leg and taken a "true-cut" biopsy, actually four small pieces, which they would send to the lab. He would call us with the results when they were ready.

At one point in the conversation, Dr. Lewis said that we would be getting the best care available anywhere. "But," he quickly added, "so does the little old lady from the Bronx." That was good; it was fine with me.

Before we left, Barry asked the doctor, "If this is a sarcoma, is there anything you can do for me?" I will never forget the answer:

"Yes, there are many things we can do," Dr. Lewis said with confidence, giving us hope. Hope.

By this time, it was quite late and many of the nurses and secretaries working at Sloan-Kettering had left for the day. I remember being impressed with how late Dr. Lewis was staying to take care of us. He didn't even know us; we had been squeezed in for a late-day appointment. At the end of our visit, it was almost dark outside, because the examination had taken so long, and then the biopsy had taken time, not to mention the time for the radiologists to examine my husband's scans. But Dr. Lewis was so dedicated that he hardly seemed to notice that he wasn't getting home when he should have. Barry and I left Sloan dazed, but with hope. At that point, my husband couldn't walk very far, and the biopsy had made him feel unsteady on his feet, so I left him at the door to Sloan in a wheel chair, with the kindly doorman looking after him, and walked the few blocks to the parking garage to get the car. Then we headed home.

CHAPTER THREE

PREPARING FOR SURGERY

In the days following our visit to Sloan-Kettering, Barry's condition deteriorated. This was to be expected, he said, after the biopsy, which had disturbed things in his leg. By now he could barely walk; he had had to stop working. I told the secretaries in his office to postpone all the appointments. I would tell them when to reschedule, as soon as I had more information. I stopped by the office daily to check things out.

By the time Dr. Lewis called a few days later with the biopsy results, Barry was hardly able to get out of bed. I was bringing all his meals to him there. Dr. Lewis gave us the bad news: the tests showed the lump to be sarcoma after all. Our worst fears were confirmed. The doctor scheduled surgery as soon as possible. The date was about a week away. I remember that he asked Barry how he was getting around, and my husband replied, "Well, I'm not, really."

When Dr. Lewis ascertained the pain Barry was having, he wanted to help. He said he could prescribe a pain-killer, just for the period before the surgery. I remember an evening phone call with him, while he was still in his office, when he said he would phone a prescription to a local pharmacy for us. I had to call around to find a pharmacy that was still open, and then call him back on his private office line. He graciously called the local drug store, and then I was able to drive over and pick up a medication that would provide some relief for us. Dr. Lewis wasn't content to just sit by and wait for a patient to ask for help; he offered it readily. But he didn't hide the truth, either. He told us that it wasn't the cancer causing the pain; it was the hemorrhage around it. That was an effort to calm our fears, but it also was the first time anyone had said the word "cancer" to us. Even though we knew what sarcoma was, we hadn't actually spoken that dreaded word, "cancer," aloud.

Now we had a short time to prepare for what we thought was "the end." Barry didn't want to leave what he considered "a mess" behind for me to deal with, and tried very hard to wind up his affairs. He made lists of instructions for me on how to run the house, the heating system, the car, and the computer by myself. He tried to do many things around the house for what he thought would be the last time. I called our accountant and lawyer, to see if there was anything we should do. We called our insurance companies to see if there was anything we needed to straighten out with them. I think it was helpful, even comforting, to be doing something, rather than just sitting around and waiting for the dreaded day. Next I called all the physicians in my husband's department at our hospital, to see if they would cover his practice for a while. How long? I didn't know. Several weeks, I guessed. Everyone was extremely cordial; frankly, I was surprised and relieved at their kindness and concern.

One of our closest friends who had faced cancer herself several years earlier told me that a good way to deal with this illness was to "compartmentalize." Just do today what has to be done today. Then tomorrow, do just what has to be done then. Trying to keep the big picture in your mind was too much, and not necessary either. That strategy really helped; it lowered the stress level somewhat. Another angel.

Our two grown daughters were extremely upset, naturally, and while I wanted to protect them, I knew they deserved to be told everything. Their stable parents, their security, were crumbling. But our daughters were wonderful, and showed remarkable strength. I felt a lot of love and support. As a family, we had had our ups and downs, but we had never faced anything like this before. I also began mentally planning my life as a caretaker, getting ready for the possibility of taking care of an invalid, a person with one leg, or even the possibility of becoming a widow. But I believed in being positive, and wouldn't stop hoping for the best until they told me it was absolutely hopeless. And maybe not then, either.

During this period, as we were trying to prepare for our uncertain future, a strange thing became clear to me. I had always assumed that someone's "self" was the physical body; now I began to feel that this was not the case at all. It seemed that the mind or personality was the real person, because as long as the mind was there, was available, then the person would be "there." While Barry could hardly get around any more, at least not without considerable pain, as long as I could ask his opinion, I still had him with me. As I contemplated not having him here any more at all, the difference between having his mind and not having his mind loomed huge. The physical capacities were not as important. This was a revelation I would never have understood previously.

Meanwhile, there were tests and scans to be performed prior to the surgery; these would be done at our local hospital, where Barry was on the staff. When I took him to have these done, since he couldn't walk any distance, I had to push him in a wheelchair through the hospital corridors in full view of his colleagues. That was hard for him. There were several doctors who couldn't take the sight of him in a wheelchair, and turned absolutely pale when they saw us. I recall Barry saying to me, after one of these men had passed us in the hall, "Well, I guess he thinks I'm a goner." I made some sort of joke, but it was grim. Then, on the way home, the night before the surgery, we stopped at Carvel for a treat. Why not? We amazed ourselves; we could still have fun. It was great to do something normal.

At some point during this period, I went to my karate school and said good-bye. I had been studying at the school for years. I told my Sensei that I would be back, but I didn't know when. It all depended on my husband's condition after the surgery, and on his recuperation. I envisioned myself taking care of a man with one leg, and not being able to leave him alone in the house. I tried to figure out how I would go shopping for food and necessities. Karate was pretty far down on the list, even though I knew it was good for my mental and physical well-being.

CHAPTER FOUR

THE LAST DAY

Two days before the surgery, amid all our preparations, Barry suddenly turned to me and said softly, "Nan, don't abandon me." It wasn't a question; it wasn't an order; it was a plea. What pain and fear he must have been feeling. *How could Barry have ever thought I would abandon him? I didn't understand it, but I did know that he needed me to assure him that I would be there.*

We got up very early on the morning of the admission to the hospital, the day before the surgery. We planned to drive down to Memorial Sloan-Kettering before the rush hour. I had made this drive before; I knew the way. Frankly, the main concern I had was how to get Barry down the stairs in the house, out to the garage, and into the car. He was in considerable pain by now, and walking just that short distance would be difficult.

As we were getting ready, we got a phone call from a nurse in Dr. Lewis's office, asking if we could get down to NYC earlier than previously scheduled. They wanted us there as soon as we could get there. We dropped everything, and got dressed as quickly as we could, without time to worry about the logistics of the stairs. As it turned out, Barry walked downstairs, then rested on a couch in the family room for a short while; then he was able to make it out to the car. But he couldn't sit upright, since that put too much pressure on the underside of his thigh. We rigged up a small carton under his foot on the floor of the car, which elevated his leg so that his thigh was off the seat. That would do for the hour's drive we had to make. I remember looking around as I drove through our small town towards the highway, thinking to myself that I didn't know when or how I would return. *By myself? With my husband? Would he ever come home? Was this the last time we would drive this road together?*

Once we arrived at Sloan-Kettering, I dropped Barry off at the front door of the hospital, and, since they were accustomed to dealing with people in his condition, they easily helped him into a wheel chair while I parked the car in a parking garage nearby, connected by an underground passageway to the hospital itself. I felt as if we had stepped onto a conveyor belt into the unknown. But there was a measure of comfort in being in competent hands.

There was a lot of paperwork for me to do in the admissions department, and, luckily, I had brought all the appropriate forms, such as Barry's Living Will and Health Care Proxy. Not so long ago, these papers had seemed like things for other people, not for healthy people like us. I also had a small bag with me, which I had packed with what I considered necessities: my address book with emergency numbers and ways to reach everyone important to me, and a change of clothes, just in case.

Eventually, we were led upstairs to a hospital floor, but since a room was not ready for us yet, we had to wait in the family lounge. It's unnerving to be processed through a system like MSKCC; you feel as if you have totally lost control; you do what you are told, by people who are at home in this environment that is so strange to you. This was the first time my husband, a physician himself, had ever been a patient. He had never been in this position in his entire life. That itself was hard to believe. Imagine being used to giving the orders, taking care of patients and their families, doing the surgery, and then finding yourself in the condition of the helpless, dependent patient. And, on top of that, not knowing whether or not you would survive.

Later that day, settled in the hospital room, Barry and I looked around, and tried to absorb it all. This would be our new home; we didn't know that it would be for only a week. While nurses and technicians performed tests on my husband, taking him to other areas of the hospital, I tried to relax downstairs in the cafeteria. I couldn't help staring at all the other people there, and wondering about their stories. Some were family members, going through exactly what I was, and others were obviously hospital staff, just as my husband had been a few weeks earlier at our local hospital.

The operation had been squeezed into the surgeon's busy schedule, and was supposed to take place at the end of the next surgical day. I had planned on going home that night and returning the next day, hoping to spend the night after the surgery at the home of my uncle in New York City. In the afternoon, however, we got a call in the hospital room from Dr. Lewis, saying that the surgery had been moved up. He had had a cancellation in his schedule, and he would now be able to operate on Barry first thing in the morning. That was good news. But it meant that I would have to be at the hospital by 7:30 AM. Perhaps I could change my plans and stay overnight at my uncle's that evening, so I could get back to the hospital easily the next morning. When I called my uncle, he said of course it was okay. I now realize how hard this was for him and his new wife. He had lost his first wife several years earlier to cancer, and our situation brought up painful memories for him.

Our older daughter, Ellen, lived and worked in Manhattan, and she came to Sloan-Kettering to meet me after work. It was comforting to see her, and I felt lucky to have her with me. I'm sure that Barry felt the same. There wasn't much to say; we all were so worried, but just being together was fine. Ellen is an artistic person, not a scientist, and tends to shy away from medical situations. We laughed as she began to feel faint and had to lie down. When dinner time neared, she and I kissed Barry good-night and headed for the door, leaving our patient in the hands of the nurses on the floor, none of us knowing what tomorrow would bring.

My daughter and I traveled the short distance to my uncle's apartment, and he and his new wife were kind enough to take us out to dinner. I had felt sure I wouldn't be able to eat anything, but agreed to accompany them just to be polite. We strolled through the warm evening air a few blocks to their favorite local restaurant, and, I must admit, they did distract me from my worries. I actually had my mind on other things for a while. And to my surprise I did eat dinner. Although Ellen offered to stay overnight with me, it really wasn't necessary, and I wanted her to do what she had planned for the evening. I wanted to be by myself, to feel myself in my new role. As we returned to my uncle's apartment, he quietly asked the doorman to call a taxi for Ellen; then he gave her money for the cab. Not realizing what he had done, I gave her taxi money as well. After she left, we laughed, realizing what had happened, saying that she probably took the taxi to the nearest subway, and pocketed the two taxi fares.

I did fall asleep that night; I don't know how. I hadn't slept in the city for many years. The noises and lights were reminiscent of my childhood, and for the first time in a very long time, I slept alone. But so did my husband, a few blocks away.

CHAPTER FIVE

THE SURGERY

I enjoyed my solitary walk to Sloan-Kettering early the next morning; it took about half an hour at a leisurely pace. I had plenty of time, and was not in a rush. I had a lot on my mind, and I didn't mind letting it all simmer in my head, without focusing on any one detail. The city was waking up at that hour, and I relished the life going on around me: the kids being walked to school, the doormen hosing down the sidewalks in front of their buildings, and the shops opening up for breakfast customers. It was wonderful to see people in their daily routines, doing normal things. Years ago, I had been a teacher here, and had begun my days like this, walking through the city streets.

When I reached the hospital, my job was to check in and then wait in the area of the lobby designated for families. Everybody sitting here had a loved one upstairs in an operating room. A million stories. Each patient belonged to a concerned person waiting. I ventured to the cafeteria, but could only eat a chocolate chip cookie. Comfort food. I had already learned about that. Shortly, Ellen joined me, and we waited together. Barry's surgery had already started; it would be about four or five hours before it was over.

Memorial Sloan-Kettering has a practice of letting waiting families know how the surgery is progressing. This is extremely kind. From time to time, the receptionist would call out a patient's name, and a family member would go to a telephone to receive word from a nurse or doctor. This way, you were not kept in the dark during the entire operation, which could take hours.

I was called to the phone several times. First I spoke to the nurse, who told me that all was going well, and that the doctor was pleased. This sort of information is invaluable to those waiting in suspense, with only their imaginations for comfort. Finally, the voice on the other end of the phone was that of Dr. Lewis, with his familiar accent.

He said that the tumor was out and all looked good so far. He told me they would call me to the recovery room shortly, but that in the meantime I should meet him in his office in ten minutes. I should bring along anyone I had with me.

By this time, Ellen and I had been joined by my brother, Bruce, and his wife, Jane, who had driven through the night from their home in Charlottesville, Va. I hadn't thought it would be necessary for them to come, but they insisted, and now I appreciated it.

The four of us made our way through the maze of corridors and elevators, up to the offices on the eleventh floor, and met Dr. Lewis. He was his usual self: energetic, warm, comforting. He explained that the surgery had gone well; they had removed the tumor completely, although it had been large (ten cm). He thought he had gotten "clean margins," but microscopic examination would be the final test of that. They had removed a large vein, and reconstructed another one, after removing a section of it. The large muscle on the inner thigh, the gracilis, was now gone, as were portions of some other muscles and a large nerve. Barry would have no feeling in a section of his leg permanently. The doctor tried to anticipate what would happen during the next week for us, and the condition Barry would be in when I brought him home. We all listened intently, trying to remember everything. My brother is a physician, so I felt confident in his ability to anticipate problems as well. Dr. Lewis said that his first priority was to save my husband's life; the second was to save his leg. And there was still a danger of infection.

I remember asking Dr. Lewis about our daughter, Sara, who now lived in Alaska, coming to visit: did she need to come in right away, or could she wait until Thanksgiving, two months away? He said she could wait; then I asked whether she could wait until the Christmas vacation, when she would be able to stay longer. She could wait until then, he said. Barry would live at least until the end of December. Dr. Lewis knew exactly what I was asking him.

Before we left the office, Dr. Lewis turned to each one of us individually, asking if we had any questions. He always ended his visits with a summary of the important facts, to help us pull the ideas together. We thanked him, and he left to prepare for his next operation. The rest of us stood in the hallway, still numb, reviewing the details. Shortly, Dr. Lewis emerged from another office, walking briskly towards the operating room, and was surprised to see us still standing outside his office. He offered to show us to the elevator, thinking that we were lost, but we were just lingering, mulling over the facts, and trying to sort things out.

Back in the waiting area, I heard my name called to go to the recovery room. I think I was supposed to go alone, but Ellen wanted to accompany me. We all knew that this would be a bad idea. She was prone to feeling faint in medical situations, and surely would be nervous at seeing her father just coming out of anesthesia. But she was adamant; I couldn't persuade her not to come upstairs. Finally my sister-in-law chimed in, echoing my position, and Ellen relented. I understood my daughter's concern, and appreciated that she wanted to be supportive, but I still thought it would be better if I went alone. So I marched after the volunteer by myself as she led me back upstairs and through more doors and down more corridors. The recovery room was large, and Barry was lying on one of the beds. The first thing I did was look down at his feet; I could see two of them sticking up under the sheets! That was a miracle.

Barry was still groggy and I began to feel a little faint myself, looking at him lying in the hospital bed after the stress of the morning. One of the nurses brought me a chair and a drink of water; I guess they were used to visitors getting woozy. Barry was able to talk a little, and soon a young anesthesiologist came over and introduced herself. She had been his anesthetist, and talked to us for a minute or two.

Barry was having trouble understanding that his surgery was over. Time had stood still for him; he didn't realize that five or six hours had passed since the doctor had started to give him anesthesia. The last thing he remembered was this young woman asking him, prior to the surgery, if he would like something to help him relax. The next thing Barry knew, a nurse was telling him that his surgery was over. He couldn't understand how it could have been finished so quickly, and kept saying, "Whose surgery is over?"

By then it was time for me to leave the recovery room, and I found my way back to the waiting area and my family. The surgery was over; it had been successful. A miracle. At times like this, I felt so grateful that there were such dedicated doctors and nurses in the world.

CHAPTER SIX

THE HOSPITAL STAY

We were amazed at how good Barry looked when we visited with him upstairs in his hospital room later in the day. He was comfortable and cheerful. He told me later that he had been extremely apprehensive before the surgery, since, as a surgeon himself, he knew all the risks involved, especially regarding anesthesia. He had been imagining all sorts of nightmarish scenarios, such as the anesthesia paralyzing him so he couldn't communicate, but not putting him under so he wouldn't feel anything. Well, at least it was over.

Now, resting in the hospital bed, Barry was hooked up to all sorts of appliances. He had an IV in, but also there was a drainage tube and bottle at the site of the surgery, and a cuff of sorts around his good leg, which inflated and deflated periodically to stimulate blood flow. He had a morphine drip for pain, and a device that allowed him to increase the pain medication at will. Actually, he never needed to use the morphine at all. I guessed that this was partly because a nerve had been removed from his leg, and he had no feeling there.

Barry's condition was remarkable; we were so lucky. Not so his hospital roommate, a man of about fifty, who had just learned that he had only months to live. The surgeons had opened him up, only to discover that there was nothing they could do for him. He had friends there constantly, trying to comfort him, saying that they would make these last months good ones for him. This poor man was clearly agitated, and kept his television on twenty-four hours a day to distract him from his thoughts; understandable, but nevertheless difficult for Barry to live with. From the window in our hospital room, you could see the East River and Welfare Island with the tram running across to it, and the 59th Street Bridge; what a marvelous sight it all would have been had the circumstances been different.

Ellen, Bruce, Jane and I ate dinner that evening downstairs in the Sloan-Kettering cafeteria; this was to be one of many meals we had there. Somehow it was comforting to be eating with the other families of patients. Before we left Barry that evening, we made a list of the phone numbers he wanted to have at hand: numbers he might not have in his head, such as family in the city, their work and home numbers. My husband kept that slip of paper next to his bedside for years.

After dinner we said good-bye, left the hospital, and we all made our way home to my house. I hadn't been home in two days. It felt like an eternity since I had closed the door to my home the day before.

Inside the house, the answering machine was flashing furiously. I was suddenly exhausted; I didn't even have the energy to pay attention to the messages. My family kindly listened to them and answered some of the phone calls coming in. It seemed that many people were waiting to hear the news. This had all been especially hard on my mother, who, as she grew older, had come to rely on Barry and me for so much. I told her how well everything had gone, trying to alleviate her worry. I was actually getting hoarse from speaking to all the concerned friends and relatives. We dealt with all we could. I remember sitting on the couch in a daze, saying aloud, "I'm home. And I'm not a widow." We all went to bed early.

Before returning to Sloan-Kettering the next morning, I had to stop at our local hospital and pick up a copy of x-rays we had had taken just before the surgery. As I walked down the familiar hallway, I encountered two of Barry's colleagues. One of them was the doctor who turned pale each time he saw my husband; now he did the same with me. He had been smiling when I approached the area, but as soon as he saw me, his face fell and he looked like he wanted to run away. I was determined not to let this attitude get to me. "Hi," I greeted him, "Don't look so glum. Everything is going very well; the surgery was a success." He stammered and said that this was just too close to him. The other doctor walked with me to the x-ray department and was very solicitous. I guess some of us are able to deal with people in crises, and some are not.

That day, back at Memorial Sloan-Kettering, Barry looked great. He was able to sit up in a chair, was eating, had good color, and was in good spirits. I think part of this was due to his general good health and the fact that he had exercised for years, swimming almost every day. I guess that a good part of it was due to the skill of the surgeon. That surgeon: our savior. He visited Barry's room a lot during the next several days, always concerned and always encouraging. Later, when I tried to express my thanks to him for the success of the surgery, he said, "It's not me; it's The Man Upstairs."

Before we knew it, the staff had Barry up and walking the hospital corridors. We saw many other patients doing the same, each shuffling along, pushing his IV pole on wheels. Each trying to get exercise, to make it back. Each determined. I felt as if we were part of a parade of walking wounded, every one hoping against all odds that he would be the one to make it.

And so the next five days passed. Doctors and residents visiting and examining Barry's leg; nurses checking his vital signs, changing his dressings; physical therapists working with him. Every day Barry was stronger; when we walked the hallway, he even lifted his walker up in the air now and then, trying to be funny. One day, our surgeon's nurse came up behind us as we were walking, surprised at my husband's energy. "Is that our patient?" we heard, in her British accent. She was hardly able to believe that he was moving so fast. One of the last things the physical therapist taught Barry was how to go up and down stairs with a cane. Then he was ready to go home.

I know this sounds strange, but I had come to love Sloan-Kettering. I found that every person we had encountered in that hospital was compassionate and kind, from the doctors down to the janitors. Every single person. Nobody was too busy to greet you with a smile and a cheerful, "Good morning." Of course, there were individual differences, but, by and large, the staff really made a difficult time much better, and made us feel less alone. Barry especially enjoyed the early morning visits of the elderly janitor, a man of particular good cheer, who greeted him with a smile every morning, as he emptied the waste baskets. I bet this man never dreamed how much his good natured greeting meant to the patients.

By now, my brother and his wife had to return home to Virginia, and Ellen had let me stay alone overnight in my house. It was exhausting for her to come home every night with me, just to rush back into the city early the following morning for work. I got used to driving back and forth myself, past Yankee Stadium and the World Series crowds; one day I got stuck in the middle of the stadium traffic. Somehow, I found that comforting, too; I was part of a large group of good-natured drivers, all stuck in the same situation. I felt part of humanity.

Shortly before discharge, a young surgeon, an oncology fellow who had appeared with Dr. Lewis during several of the examinations, came into Barry's hospital room. He had stopped by several times to see how the healing was progressing, and could identify with my husband, since they both had been surgery residents. He seemed pleased with the progress, and when he left, he said good-bye and wished my husband good luck. I'll never forget him saying, "Don't come back here." A sweet man, but a grim reminder that many patients did indeed return to Sloan-Kettering.

On the day of Barry's discharge, Ellen met me at the hospital to help with the trip home. I had expected to need assistance getting him into the house, and had almost asked some neighbors if they could help me with the wheel chair I had been sure we would need. I had planned on having to live downstairs for a while until Barry was able to negotiate the steps upstairs. However, my proud husband walked slowly inside, and up the stairs to the living room himself. I was glad that Ellen was there to see her father's strength and determination.

We were home together, but everything was different. I knew that Barry had thought he might never see this place again. We had both wondered if he would ever sleep in our bed beside me again; how very wonderful it was to have him back.

CHAPTER SEVEN

AT HOME
(Sept - Oct '98)

We spent the next few days getting adjusted to the process of recuperation. We did things slowly, and took leisurely walks back and forth along the quiet road in front of our house, with Barry leaning on his cane. He had to depend on that cane, but did quite well; and the fresh air was great for him. A couple of friends came over to visit, and we felt a lot of support. Emotionally, we were scared, but very upbeat, and the encouragement of our surgeon helped a lot. This was new territory.

On Saturday, the fourth day after the hospital discharge, our phone rang at 7:30 in the morning. When I answered it, I was surprised to hear Dr. Lewis's voice on the line. He was calling to ask how Barry was doing; he wanted to chat with him, to hear how he sounded. When the doctor discharged my husband, he had told him to call and check in in a few days. Barry had not done that, not wanting to bother Dr. Lewis. We learned then and there that when Dr. Lewis asked you to call him, he meant it!

Meanwhile, I was trying to do as many "normal" things as possible, which was the advice of friends who had lived through this kind of thing themselves. I went to the dentist, got a flu shot, and even went swimming, as had been my old habit. It was really nice to feel the warmth of the people I encountered, many of whom were very concerned, and very kind. When I stopped in at our own office, which I did daily, invariably I found messages or notes from concerned patients or colleagues. I was amazed; I guess I had been cynical about things like this in the past. I now believed that people really did care, but wouldn't necessarily show it unless they thought you needed to hear it. So if you appeared to be strong or independent, you might never know that people cared.

We began to talk about going back to work again, and planned to open office hours in a couple of weeks. Our secretaries started rescheduling all the appointments they had cancelled. First we had to see Barry's surgeon again, and we also scheduled a visit with a radiology oncologist, who would plan the radiation needed to prevent the tumor from recurring in Barry's leg. Slowly, we edged back into life; not the old life, but a new life. But any life was okay with me.

The week after the hospital discharge, just two weeks after the surgery, it was our thirty-third wedding anniversary. That was the day we had an appointment with Dr. Lewis down at Sloan-Kettering. Before he had gone in for surgery, Barry had given me an anniversary card. He thought he might not be around to give it to me later.

At MSKCC, Dr. Lewis again was upbeat, encouraging us to be positive. He thought Barry looked very good. He always had people he was teaching with him: medical students, residents, or fellows. This time two young women were in the room, and when it was time for my husband's stitches to be removed, Dr. Lewis instructed them to do it. There were many, many stitches, extending from his knee all the way up to his groin. The nurses were tentative, but taking out stitches is not hard, and all went well.

There was one more procedure to be performed during the exam: Dr. Lewis had to remove a staple from my husband's backside. A few days before this, Barry had felt something bothering him when he sat down, and asked me if there was anything strange there. I took a look: *could that be a staple?* I told him that it looked like a staple, but I couldn't believe it. He laughed; being a surgeon, he knew that "these things happen," and was amused that, after performing hours of delicate and complicated surgery, Dr. Lewis's team had neglected to remove the last staple from his body. I couldn't imagine what a staple had been doing in Barry's body anyway, but he told me that it had probably been used to hold a tube in place during the operation. When we told Dr. Lewis on the telephone what we had found, he had said that he would take it out when we came down to see him. Now, at the visit, he had to pull out the offending staple. He did it without using any anesthetic. This was no piece of cake: Barry said it hurt like crazy. But it still was funny. A sense of humor didn't hurt at times like this.

Dr. Lewis then told us about the plans for radiation. The treatments would not be difficult to handle, he said. They were not painful, and didn't cause discomfort except for some fatigue after a few weeks. Dr. Lewis would keep in touch with us frequently, for support. When my husband asked him whether he thought we would be able to keep our office open, he answered, "Of course." He thought it was good for Barry to start working again. And not to hide the fact that he had cancer, either. *How would we handle that, we wondered? How would our patients deal with it? Who would still come to a doctor who had a dreaded disease?* Dr. Lewis was calm, repeating that he thought we should not hide Barry's condition. At any rate, we knew that it would be difficult, if not impossible, to hide it. So we decided to be candid about it, and see what happened. And we knew it was the right thing to do, for if more of us were honest about cancer, then people might stop avoiding those who had it.

Several days later, Barry asked me to look at his leg; way up at the top of the incision something felt strange. I looked, and, sure enough, way at the top, the nurses had left a stitch in, and it was irritating him. It would be up to me to take it out. I am not a trained medical person, and even though I had taken out stitches once before, I was very nervous about doing it this time, since this was the site of major surgery. But my husband couldn't see this area, much less reach it and manipulate the tools himself. He didn't want to bother any of the local doctors, either, and going all the way down to Memorial Sloan-Kettering for this was silly. So I gritted my teeth and did it. I needed a magnifier, a pair of scissors, and tweezers. When I looked closely, I saw that the skin had started growing over the stitch; I would have to pull the stitch up with the tweezers, and try to cut it without cutting my husband's skin. I didn't like this one bit, but somehow, I managed to do the job.

CHAPTER EIGHT

GETTING READY FOR RADIATION

One rainy autumn afternoon, we made the thirty-five minute drive to Phelps Hospital in Sleepy Hollow, the location of MSKCC's Westchester site for radiation and chemotherapy. Barry walked into the building, using his cane. Again we were on unfamiliar ground, surrounded by nurses, technicians and doctors who dealt daily with cancer. And recurrences. Old people, young people, every patient here had cancer. The waiting room was composed of little booths for privacy; patients and families could wait or consult in relative quiet.

There were snacks and drinks provided and a wonderful, large fish tank with brightly colored fish swimming back and forth. How we enjoyed those fish! We got to know every one of them and their habits: which ones hid among the seaweed, which ones chased the others around. They were beautiful; their colors and shapes were amazing; some were iridescent, some dull, some round and fat, some paper-thin. But it was surprising to see how each displayed its distinctive personality. Who would ever believe that a fish tank could give patients so much enjoyment? Somehow it was a calming influence. We found out that some of the technicians even came in on the week-ends to check the fish or feed them.

Our first appointment was with the radiology-oncologist, Dr. M., who was to direct Barry's course of treatment. The purpose of the treatments was to prevent a local recurrence, that is, in his leg. The radiation would consist of daily doses which would last only a few minutes, and the treatments would continue for about eight weeks. The area to be radiated was the upper leg, a section from just above the knee clear up to the pubic bone, the length of the surgery site. The radiation would eventually make the leg tissue hard, like wood, and the skin would become extremely dark, dry and leathery.

Before the treatments could start, there were several long preparatory appointments. The technicians had to make a cast for Barry to place his leg in during the radiation, and many x-rays were taken and measurements made. We met and consulted with the head technician, an outgoing woman with long, gray hair streaming down her back. She was a master at what she did, not only of the technical side, but also the psychological. She was a real character, very dedicated, very competent, with a great sense of humor; she was also a little fearsome. A no-nonsense kind of person. We also met Dr. M.'s nurse, another compassionate soul, who gave us lots of information about how best to deal with side effects, which were not so much debilitating as inconvenient. We found that all of the young technicians who worked there were exceptional people: kind, gentle, and always willing to laugh. That really helped.

The radiation room was awesome: eerie, and more than a little frightening. It was a very large, white space, with a lonely table in the middle, over which stood a huge radiation machine. This machine could rotate around the table, so that radiation could be directed at the patient from all angles. There were red laser beams which emanated from holes in the walls of the room, to guide the technicians in placement of the patient. And, strangely, the technicians would have to tattoo dots on the radiation field of Barry's leg, to line up with those red beams. When they were finished with the positioning, everyone would hurry out of the room, leaving my husband, the solitary patient, alone on the huge table, ready for the radiation poison.

One day, the technicians let me come in and watch the radiation, instead of sitting in the waiting area. I stood with them just outside the radiation room, watching two television screens, and could see Barry lying on the table in the middle of this huge room. There were two cameras trained on him. Two, just in case something happened to one. They couldn't take any chances here. He looked small in the large, spotlessly white space. It looked like something out of science fiction, but with my husband in the scene. Odd as all this felt at first, the human mind is adaptable, and very quickly it all became routine.

The first day that Barry received treatment was the last day of treatment for a young college girl. She had the same kind of rare tumor, only hers had been even larger than my husband's. The young woman's parents sat waiting for her, holding flowers, while she completed the last session of her months of radiation. It was startling to be talking to a family who were finishing up with the long course we were just beginning. I hadn't dared to think that far ahead. When they left, they kissed me and wished us well. Dealing with this sort of trouble created a bond between people.

CHAPTER NINE

RETURNING TO WORK AND ROUTINE

We completed all the preparatory appointments for the radiation, and before the treatments started, Barry returned to working in his office. He couldn't be on his feet for a whole day because his leg was prone to swelling due to the loss of a big vein from the surgery. We decided to work just in the mornings. But at least we were back in our office; another step into "normalcy."

The office had not been closed for long - just a few weeks during the surgery and recuperation - but it seemed like eons to us. Many of our patients didn't know anything had happened. Others, who knew us better, or whose appointments had been postponed, did know. I was astounded by their reactions. Every patient without exception offered support. Some had been praying for us; others had sent cards or brought cookies. Several patients cried when they heard our story. I began to feel like the luckiest person alive. I would never have known about all the good feelings people had for us, if it hadn't been for the strange tragedy of this cancer.

Once the radiation treatments started, our routine was set: work in the morning, a small picnic lunch in the office, and then over to the Sloan-Kettering facility at Phelps Hospital for the treatments. When Barry was admitted into the radiation room, the treatment didn't last long. We would spend an hour or two there. We saw the same patients day after day. I had my own strategy for making the time pass in the waiting area: I brought books, magazines, and my drawing supplies. It was my quiet time, time for myself, time for my mind to wander, and time to be renewed.

About three months after Barry's surgery, I resumed my morning swim on the days that Barry felt up to driving himself to the office. I also had enough energy to return to karate class, which was important "for my head." This refreshed my spirit, and gave me something else to focus on.

Each day, as we approached Phelps Hospital, we noticed a parking area with room for just five or six cars, and often saw a few people walking up a path. We had no idea where this led, but we were curious. One day we had a little time before our appointment, so we decided to park the car and follow the path. It led up a hill. The climb was difficult for Barry to negotiate, but I thought the exercise would be good for him.

The path headed west, and at the top of the hill a magnificent view unfolded in front of us: between the trees we saw the Hudson River stretching out below, with the broad expanse of the cliffs of the Palisades on the other side. We were breathless! From that day on, we made time to walk in this glorious park every day before the radiation. This infused a sense of peace into our daily routine. It slowed us down and invited us to take in the beautiful surroundings. We came to love this walk with its various paths, and to enjoy the change of seasons there: fall would become winter during the course of the radiation. We loved the huge, gnarled, trees, the oaks and weeping beeches growing there. Occasionally we saw deer. The walkways were old carriage paths left over from the days when this had been a Rockefeller estate. What a setting for a home this must have been. And what a wonderful interlude it became in our daily lives, slipped in between our work in the office and Barry's radiation treatments.

During the months following Barry's discharge from Sloan-Kettering, we checked in with Dr. Lewis by phone weekly. He had asked us to call him, and it became a welcome routine for us. Dr. Lewis was always encouraging, and gradually we came to rely on his cheerful optimism for a little "pick-me-up." How he had the time for us in his hectic days, I will never know, since in addition to his full surgical schedule, he had office hours, and was engaged in ongoing cancer research. Dr. Lewis had so much to give, and we felt lucky to have found him. I have never in my life met anyone so generous with his time and spirit. Once in a while, he would ask Barry questions which revealed an unexpected curiosity, such as, "What's it like for you to be a patient?" Dr. Lewis wanted to know about everything, and Barry could tell him about the situation from a perspective Dr. Lewis didn't have. How many physicians ask questions like these? How many care to know this much?

CHAPTER TEN

AUTUMN
(Nov '98)

It was fall, and when Halloween rolled around, all the technicians at the radiation facility wore costumes. They were young and energetic people; their cheerfulness made this treatment easier to handle. I couldn't understand what had made them choose this profession that seemed so grim to me, but I was thankful they had and were so kind. They seemed to love their work. One of the young men was dressed up for the day to look like his boss, the head technician. He had on a long gray wig, a dress, and make-up. What a character!

October turned to November, and we were involved in the daily business of work and radiation, trying hard to include some treats, such as exercise, peaceful walks, and dinners out with friends. We developed a balance in our lives that was essential in this situation, and really belongs in every situation. In addition to attending to Barry, I learned how to take care of myself mentally and emotionally. *If you don't take the time to restore yourself spiritually, you are no good to anyone.*

In early November, my cousins planned a 50th wedding celebration for my aunt and uncle in California. As a very young child, I had been the flower girl at their wedding, and they had always been special to me. My aunt is my mother's younger sister, and the two of them were extremely close, often living near each other, and at one time during my childhood living next door to each other. But my aunt and uncle had moved to California about five years before this to be near their children and grandchildren. This meant the first long-distance separation for my mother and her sister, and it was hard on both of them. Now my cousins were taking the occasion of their parents' 50th anniversary to throw a family party for a lot of people who hadn't seen each other in some time. Everyone was looking forward to it.

The only shadow cast on the celebration was Barry's illness. As the date neared, I tried to figure out a way that we could attend. We had radiation every day, and we didn't want to jeopardize the effectiveness of the treatment by missing sessions. On the other hand, the nurses were encouraging us to lead as normal a life as possible, and they knew that special occasions and celebrations were good for patients and their families. Going to the party would mean a quick cross-country trip to California, which was a strenuous undertaking. I wasn't sure that Barry had the endurance for such a trip, and I didn't know how long he could sit on a plane without real discomfort. The physical cost seemed too high. We would miss two radiation treatments, and if there were delays, we would miss more. There didn't seem any way to work it out. Barry and I had an unspoken understanding: *I wouldn't consider leaving him and going myself; it was out of the question.* So, with a good deal of sadness, I told my aunt and uncle that we just couldn't join them. They understood. We sent flowers; the family sent us photos of the party afterwards, but it was disappointing. We would visit them as soon as we could travel. That was a promise.

It was also during November that Barry developed sciatica. It was acutely painful, and sent spasms down his leg. He had pulled his back while trying to start a leaf-blower. (He was always doing whatever he could around the house; he hated to feel like an invalid.) The sciatica set back his recuperation. He had to cancel his work schedule for a few days; standing and sitting became too painful for him. But we didn't miss any radiation treatments! I remember his pain as we made our daily drive to the hospital. He couldn't sit upright in the car; he had to stretch out any way he could in order to make it bearable. But with time, this, too, passed, and it was just another bump in the road to recovery.

When Thanksgiving came, we had the family party at our house as usual; I wanted desperately to continue our tradition. I kept the preparations as simple as possible, and it worked out well: everyone in our family was much more interested in getting together than in how fancy the food was. This was indeed another miracle. Some of the family expressed surprise that we undertook the job, but I needed things to feel normal.

The day after Thanksgiving, Barry had his usual radiation treatment scheduled. My mother was staying at our house for the weekend, so we had two choices: to leave her home alone for several hours, or to bring her along. We decided to take her. She is not comfortable in medical situations, but she tried hard to be strong. We took her with us on our customary short scenic walk before the session, and then she waited with me, enjoying the company of the nurses and technicians while Barry had his treatment. It was an eye-opener for her.

Illness is part of life; you cannot hide from it. Hiding only isolates you anyway, and encourages fear. It sends a signal that the thing you are hiding is terrible. I came to believe that the more open people are about illnesses like cancer, the less these issues will be dreaded and avoided. The more people see that cancer can be dealt with, the more they see that people can survive, even thrive and be happy while dealing with illness, the less people will shy away from cancer's victims. People were looking at me, and I felt that I had to show them that we were okay. I was becoming an example of how to deal with cancer.

At times, I felt hopeless or discouraged, and I remember thinking to myself, as I walked along the streets of our town looking at young, healthy people, that they couldn't grasp what might be in store for them. *Who knew what might be growing inside their own bodies at any given moment? Who would have guessed, looking at my husband the day before the lump appeared in his leg, what was lurking in his body?*

CHAPTER ELEVEN

THE HOLIDAYS
(Dec '98)

With only a few weeks of radiation left, we were scheduled for an appointment with our surgeon, Dr. Lewis, down at Memorial Sloan-Kettering Cancer Center. By now, Barry was hardly using his cane and we were proud of his recuperation. The doctor thought Barry looked very good. We were hopeful as we approached the end of the radiation treatments.

Dr. Lewis had a story to tell us. His department at Sloan-Kettering had received an email message from a man in Cleveland who had had sarcoma thirty years ago, and had been treated at the hospital. The man had had surgery and radiation, and then returned home to Cleveland. Thirty years ago! The reason that this man had emailed Sloan that fall was that the Yankees had just won the World Series against Cleveland, and he remembered that when he had been a patient in Sloan thirty years ago, the Yankees had been playing Cleveland in the Series then, too. These two teams had not played each other in the World Series since then, and the current play-offs had reminded him of the games he had listened to on the radio in his hospital room. He wanted to let the doctors know that he was still doing well. This was Dr. Lewis's way of telling us that sarcoma patients could live.

Up to this point, we had been checking in by phone every week with Dr. Lewis. At the end of our appointment, as we were preparing to leave the examination room, he said something general about "keeping in touch." *What?* I felt like a boat which had just been unhooked from the dock, to drift and flounder in unknown waters. *Keep in touch?* We had come to rely on this wonderful man's weekly encouragement, and on his knowledge of what would happen next. I couldn't let his remark pass. I vividly recall the desperation in my heart as I asked, "Don't you want us to call you next week?" The way I blurted it out made us all laugh. I was embarrassed. I guess Dr. Lewis sensed my fear, and said with a smile, "Of course, I do."

Out in the waiting area, we lingered while the nurses scheduled our next appointment, three months hence. They told us to have a CAT scan before then, and to fax the report to Dr. Lewis. As we stood there, making the arrangements, Dr. Lewis suddenly appeared from the examining room corridor, looking for us. He had another patient in the exam room, a man who had had sarcoma in his leg, just like my husband, three years earlier. He, too, had had radiation treatments, and was doing just fine. Dr. Lewis wanted Barry to meet this patient, and see how well he was doing, so we went back into the exam area. The man, older than Barry, was indeed in great shape, able to work, exercise and enjoy life. In fact, since recovering, he was enjoying life more than ever. We ended up spending a long time talking to the man and his wife. This gave us hope: another example of life after sarcoma.

The last day of radiation was a bittersweet time. It was a relief to complete these treatments; there was no doubt of that. But we would be leaving the security of being seen at a medical facility every day. While these daily visits had been occurring, we felt that if something was wrong, the doctors and nurses would notice. Now, we were "cut loose." We would have our scans and appointments with Dr. Lewis every three months, but aside from that, we were on our own.

We didn't know it, but every patient received a diploma upon completion of the course of radiation. The technicians drew a colorful certificate, and everyone signed it with good luck wishes. The staff presented it to Barry at the end of the day. We hugged them all, and gave them gifts of chocolate. Slowly, we walked away from Phelps Hospital, finished with radiation. Another milestone.

Four days later, our younger daughter Sara and her husband Richard flew in from Alaska for the holidays. The December holidays: a season we had thought we would never share again. The young people arrived at Westchester Airport at 9 AM after traveling all night from Fairbanks, and stopping en route in Anchorage, Seattle, and Chicago. We hadn't seen them since the day after Barry's tumor first appeared, on our last visit with them in Seattle, a few weeks before they had moved to Fairbanks. What a six months it had been! But at least we were all still here to celebrate.

To say that we enjoyed the holidays that year would be an understatement. It was heaven to have Sara and Richard with us. Our daughter had so much to show her husband, who had grown up in southern California, and had never been to New York. She took him to some of her favorite places, and he had a chance to meet her friends who were home for holiday visits. We spent a wonderful couple of days, and then were joined by our daughter, Ellen, from Manhattan. It was so good to have the whole family together again! The three young people spent some time in the city, with Ellen showing the others her home territory: New York City in all its holiday splendor. Near the end of the week, the rest of our extended family arrived: my mother, and my brother, his wife, and their two adult children. This was surely a holiday to celebrate, and we all felt lucky to have each other.

Before we knew it, Sara and Richard were on the return flight to Fairbanks; their schedules didn't allow much time off. But the warmth of the visit lasted a long, long time. We continued the holiday with the rest of our family, and it wound down slowly. When everyone had left except my mother, Barry and I drove her home, ending our holidays, and knowing that the date of his next x-ray was fast approaching.

CHAPTER TWELVE

JANUARY
(1999)

January was a busy month for us. The first event was Barry's chest x-ray, scheduled for January fourth. This was the first scan to be performed after the radiation, and, naturally, we were nervous about the results. This could tell us whether the sarcoma had spread. While the surgeon had confirmed that the operation on Barry's leg had shown microscopically clean margins, we didn't know whether any cells had been released and sent rushing to other parts of his body. We did know that the most likely place for sarcoma to spread was the lungs.

You can imagine our state of mind as we waited for the x-ray report. We had the scan performed at our local hospital, and then we returned to our office across the street to await a call from the radiologist. This was the same man who had read both the first and second MRI's of Barry's leg, seven months earlier. We finally spoke to him in the afternoon; it was not his job to call patients and give them the results of x-rays, but he was doing us a favor. The report showed clean lungs! We were relieved beyond belief. Later that day, Dr. Lewis called from Sloan-Kettering to let us know that he had received the report, and was happy to tell us that Barry's lungs were clear. He, too, was enthusiastic.

Every time a cancer patient has a scan, he prepares for the worst. The results may send him back into victim mode, give him a death sentence, or may clear him to live for the next three months. It all happens with a two-minute phone call: "The test results are in." Your heart stops; you go on alert; and then you are given a green light to live again. Or not.

Now with the good report in our hands, we were ready to celebrate. Dr. Lewis told us to go on a good long vacation, and we didn't need much coaxing. For years, we had taken a trip to Arizona every February. This year, I hadn't dared to plan it until after the medical report. But we were cleared, and we were free to leave. We scheduled a three-week visit to our favorite place: northern Arizona. This would be longer than we had ever been away. And that wasn't all. We wanted to visit Sara and Richard in Alaska during the coming summer. I started planning that trip as well, since I had been told that reservations in Alaska had to be made well in advance. I was upbeat and busy, planning both trips, but with a nagging fear always in the back of my mind. *"What if....."* Lots of "what if's" would have to be resolved before we made it to Alaska in June. Meanwhile, we prepared for February in Arizona.

In the midst of all the excitement, our close friend and Barry's colleague had a heart attack and died within weeks. This was a friend who had been offering all fall to drive us over to the radiation facility. He was good-hearted and generous, and he had been eager to help. He had worked in his office next door to Barry's for years, and we had seen him daily. We were numb with disbelief. I guess we had reached that age when these things start to happen. But it always takes you by surprise. At his funeral, people were in a state of shock, and everyone seemed to be looking at Barry, amazed that he was still walking around. I kept watching our friend's wife, a new widow, knowing so well that I could have been in her shoes...

CHAPTER THIRTEEN

ARIZONA VACATION
(Feb '99)

That February, we spent three full weeks in Arizona, our favorite place. The first thing we did after arriving in Phoenix was to relax in the southwest atmosphere. We loved the western sky, the warm breezes, the birds singing, the cactus plants, the roadrunners, the smiling faces. Before we headed north to Sedona, Flagstaff and the Grand Canyon, our usual itinerary, we decided to drive to southern California to visit my aunt and uncle, whose anniversary party we had missed in the fall; we had plenty of time. They were delighted with the prospect. So we pointed our rented truck west, and drove through the desert.

Barry and I both loved hitting the road, and where better than in our favorite state? We drove out on Route 10 past little settlements, through Quartzite, the town in the middle of nowhere, that swells to many times its own size with motor homes during the winter months, over the Colorado River, past the state border and into California. We were amazed at the windmill farms outside Palm Springs as we whizzed past that little desert oasis. Before we knew it, traffic density was increasing and we were in southern California on the freeway, approaching Laguna Niguel, our destination. It was great to be free and on the open road, and to feel ourselves strong and healthy. Barry was driving and that told me how good he felt.

The visit with my relatives was a lot of fun, like old times, except that now my aunt was a cancer survivor, as was Barry. We packed a lot into that one weekend: breakfasts and dinners out, movies, strolls on the docks at Dana Point, walks along the beach with my cousins and their young children.

On Monday we said our good-byes and climbed into the truck, filled with feelings of love and support. We enjoyed the drive east towards Arizona, again making our way through the desert, stopping overnight this time. I had wanted to visit Palm Springs for a long time, but was not prepared for what we found. What a place: old folks dressed like teenagers, tourists by the hundreds, it looked like Hollywood in the desert. Then on to Arizona.

We headed for the northern part of the state, to our favorite spots: Sedona, Flagstaff, and that jewel, the Grand Canyon. Again, Barry drove; we were elated by how strong he felt. We followed our usual pattern, staying in Sedona for a few days, soaking up the warmth, hiking the trails we loved, lingering at the hilltop airport to watch the small planes taking off, and browsing the shops filled with Native American art.

When we were ready for a more rustic atmosphere, we drove up Route 89-A, making the 3000-foot climb through magnificent Oak Creek Canyon to Flagstaff. This half-hour drive is the most breathtaking I have ever seen. I never tire of it. I always kidded Barry, saying that when we retired I wanted to get a job driving the UPS truck up and down Oak Creek Canyon between Sedona and Flagstaff. In Flagstaff, we have our favorite places, too. We always visit The Museum of Northern Arizona, Bookman's Used Book Store, the historic railroad station where the Santa Fe trains lumber through, and Old Town, the historic district.

The trails in Flagstaff are often covered with snow and ice in winter, but this year the weather was warm enough for us to do some hiking. Because of the condition of Barry's leg, we chose "Fatman's Loop," a trail rated "easy" on our map. This hike was on the east side of town, and the trail wound up the side of a mountain and provided a remarkable view of the Painted Desert and the Navajo reservation; in the distance we could even make out the Hopi mesas. The trail got its name from a section that squeezes in between huge rocks, and anyone too fat simply can't fit through. About a quarter of the way into the hike, the climb became strenuous. Whoever had rated this "easy" must have been in much better shape than we were. But the beauty was worth the effort, and we took it slow to let Barry rest his leg frequently. I thought the exertion was good for him. I guess I was pushing it a bit. Along the trail, we stopped as a woman hiker pointed out a red-tailed hawk to us. On the way back down to our truck, we paused at the trailhead, and saw that, indeed, the "easy" rating on our map was wrong: the hike was clearly labeled "moderate" on the signpost!

When we visit Arizona in the winter, we never make reservations up north; we play it by ear, letting the weather determine our itinerary. We watch the forecast, and when we see two or more days ahead without snow, we head for the Grand Canyon. We know that if you call the Canyon's lodges the evening before you want to arrive you can often get a last-minute reservation. It worked that winter, too. We left Flagstaff early in the morning, and headed east on Route 40, getting off at Route 89, and driving north around the magnificent San Francisco Peaks, through the pine forests, down into the Painted Desert, and onto the Navajo Reservation. We have mandatory stops on the route. The first is at Cameron, a tiny settlement on the reservation, where the old Trading Post is a must. We love to wander around, browse through the pawned native jewelry, and buy an ice-cream. The air is warm here after the chill of the higher altitude in Flagstaff.

Then we head west on Route 64 towards Grand Canyon National Park. We stop at the Little Colorado overlook to take in views of the gorge of the Little Colorado River as it rushes to join the Colorado. But the main attraction here is the vast array of Native American goods for sale by their crafters. To me, this is the best museum around. The silver jewelry, beads, pottery, and rugs are a feast for the eyes and soul. Our trip is simply not complete without a stop here. The sun blazes down, the sky is endless blue, and the Navajo craftsmen sit with their wares, surrounded by their children. We often recognize the people, having seen them year after year. I have to tear myself away from this place, but we are on our way to The Canyon.

Approaching Grand Canyon National Park, the road climbs and the vegetation changes; soon you are surrounded by tall Ponderosa pines. The temperature drops. This time we slowed down when we saw a car stopped in the road ahead of us: they were watching a bald eagle in a tree by the side of the road. It was breathtaking, but no more a miracle than our just being there. The beauty of the place was magical for us, and I know that Barry had believed that he would never see this place again

When you enter the park, you have to buy an entry pass. Should we buy a yearly National Park pass, or just a one-time pass? Did we think we would be visiting any other national parks during the year? We decided to be optimistic and buy the annual pass; we were feeling great.

Once inside the park, we made another of our favorite stops: Desert View Overlook. From this vantage point on the Canyon's South Rim, you can see the Colorado River below, the Painted Desert to the east, and much of the Canyon as the river flows west through it. There is a gift shop, a cafe for snacks, and, of course, the Desert View Watchtower to climb. As we made our customary stops, we still did not fully believe that we were here again.

We proceeded to Grand Canyon Village with its trails, viewpoints, lodges, museums, and, finally, El Tovar, the main lodge with its magnificent lobby and fireplace. I must admit, the couch in front of the El Tovar fireplace is my favorite spot in the entire world.

CHAPTER FOURTEEN

THE GRAND CANYON

How can I describe the way I feel about the Grand Canyon? It is my religion, my cathedral, my place to contact nature's powerful forces that shaped our earth. It is so vast and so beautiful; its constantly changing moods are awesome. I have come to love it, and I need to see it, to feel it and to walk it as often as I can. It has been my greatest privilege to be able to do so.

That February, Barry and I found ourselves overwhelmed to be back at The Canyon together. While Barry had not expected to see it again, I had wondered whether I could bear to come back if I had to do it without him. But this year we had made it. We strolled along the familiar paths on the South Rim, with the canyon and all its brilliant colors right next to us. A glance over the edge brought a thrill, and we enjoyed this view for several days. We would stay as long as we wished, letting the weather be our guide.

The shops along the Canyon's rim were a pleasure for us, too. The array of Native American art is another visual "gift" for me. The native crafts, rooted in their religion and ceremonies, hold significance for me: they are in tune with nature. The Native American people do not try to control nature's forces, the way our society does. They work within her laws.

The rustic lifestyle at the Canyon always relaxes me. The people operate at a different pace from the outside world. Barry and I have a friend we have come to know because of our frequent visits, and we always look for her when we are there. She and her husband have lived and worked at the lodges for years, and it was funny when, after seeing her for a few years in a row, she suddenly said to us on one visit, "Haven't you been here before?" Since then, we always meet her. She looks for us at a certain time of year, and we find her by asking the employees which lodge she is working at that year. It is another connection we have with the place.

We spent several days immersed in the aura of the Canyon, taking photographs, walking and hiking, and being lazy by the El Tovar fireplace. Finally, when storms threatened, we headed south, back to civilization.

We drove to Flagstaff and slowly adjusted to a more "normal" pace of life. Being on vacation, we could still take our time, but it was not the same as the slow pace of life at the Canyon. We drove down Oak Creek Canyon almost every day to hike in Sedona. There are several hikes I absolutely must make, and I never get tired of the scenery. I try to imagine what it would be like to live there and to see these red rocks every day. Would you just get used to it all, and not notice after a while? On one of these hikes, we had walked deep into the forest, and were sitting on a log in a clearing, just relaxing in the sun, when some mountain bikers happened by. They asked us for directions and we chatted with them. I couldn't imagine anything more wonderful than basking in the western sun, surrounded by magnificent views, smelling the pinion pine trees, with a man whose very life was a miracle.

In Sedona that year, we spent time at Tlaquepaque, the Mexican-style shopping area in town. We had just finished browsing the art and craft stores, when we heard music, so we followed the sound. We came upon a young man playing his guitar in a courtyard. Patrick Ki, a young guitarist, had moved to Sedona from his native Hawaii, and was now the "resident musician" in the area. He spent time on the week-ends at Tlaquepaque when tourists were there, playing his compositions on the guitar accompanied by his CD's, which he sold as well. Patrick took delight in sharing his music; he seemed to be having such a good time. We purchased two CD's and sat in the afternoon sun listening to his concert. The music was ours to enjoy for as long as we cared to linger. Barry and I both felt that we were blessed that day. From then on, whenever I played these CD's at home in New York, I would be transported back to that sunny afternoon in Sedona, and smile.

As February came to an end, we had to return home, but we did so with happiness in our hearts. Barry felt good, looked great, and had been up to a lot of physical activity, something we hadn't anticipated. We flew back east with optimism for our future. We were already planning a trip to Alaska for the coming summer.

CHAPTER FIFTEEN

UNEXPECTED NEWS
(March '99)

Within a few days of our return, we were immersed in our routine with lots to do. My mother was having a cataract removed, and Barry had arranged for one of his colleagues at our local hospital to perform the surgery. I brought my mother over from New Jersey to stay at our house, and spent time with her at the office appointments, the surgery, and during the recuperation. I was with her when the anesthesiologist was explaining the procedure to her, and when he was done he asked if she had any questions. My mother looked up into the young man's eyes. "One question," she said. "Are you married?" As we collapsed in laughter, I realized that she was thinking of her unmarried granddaughter!

At the same time, we were getting ready for Barry's next check-up with Dr. Lewis at Sloan-Kettering. We were happy to see our beloved doctor again, and brought him a little gift from Arizona. He was glad to see Barry looking so well. I wanted to tell Dr. Lewis that we felt hopeful enough to plan our trip to Alaska for the coming summer. But he was so busy on that day that I didn't want to take up any extra time. But I distinctly recall his saying, in a serious tone, as we were leaving, "Be sure to get your CAT scan soon." It was nice that my husband looked good, but Dr. Lewis knew all too well that when cancer is concerned, outward appearances can belie what's going on inside. Of course, we had already scheduled the scan, and were not too worried about it.

In fact, we were so casual about the CAT scan that after it was performed, Barry and I took a walk around town, instead of waiting at our office for the radiologist to call us. I will never forget returning to the office, and hearing our secretary say, "Dr. L. called; he wants you to call him." *The radiologist certainly was calling promptly.* Without a moment's delay, my husband called him back. I stood by the desk as he spoke to the radiologist. I expected to hear, "Thanks a lot; that's good news." What I heard sent a chill through

my body. Barry's expression was grim. He kept saying, "Uh-huh
.....uh-huh.......uh-huh." Obviously, the radiologist had a lot to tell
him. When he hung up the phone, Barry's face was pale. He told me
that the CAT scan had revealed several lesions in his lungs. Several
lesions. Once again, he thought his life was over.

Events moved quickly then. Within minutes we were across
the street at the hospital, looking at the scan, while the radiologist
pointed out the lesions, in both of Barry's lungs. Though very small,
there were seven lesions. This was dire news. We waited while
the radiology department made a copy of the scan for us, and then
went back to our office. The first thing we did was call Dr. Lewis.
Fortunately, he was able to come to the phone. He told us to come
down for an appointment with him in three days, but he wanted to
see the scan in advance. Could we "Fed-Ex" it in time? Instead,
Barry and I dropped everything we were doing, drove down to
Sloan with the CAT scan in our hands, and delivered it personally
to Dr. Lewis's secretary. It had been six months since my husband's
surgery, and three months since the end of his radiation treatments.
Perfect timing for a recurrence: a metastasis to the lungs.

That Friday morning, we found ourselves in Dr. Lewis's office,
meeting with him and Dr. A., the chest surgeon he recommended. The
doctors had formulated a plan of action: heavy-duty chemo for two
months, chest surgery, and then four more months of chemo. They
called this a "heroic" plan, but they thought it had a good chance of
working. We were grateful to them for moving so quickly.

My head was spinning. Again, we were entering unknown territory;
it was like being in a black hole. Barry talked to the doctors. "I guess
this means the end of my practice." "Not at all!" was the reply from
both doctors. It would be good for my husband to keep his office open.
We couldn't for the life of us see how it could be done, but they knew
what they were talking about, and we accepted their advice. I distinctly
recall Dr. Lewis saying to us that if we did nothing at this point, Barry
could expect to live for about one more year. We never considered
avoiding the treatment, but this was sobering nonetheless.

The first thing we had to deal with was the chemotherapy.
"Chemotherapy:" the very word conjures up all sorts of terrifying

images. But once you make your decision, you forge ahead as optimistically as possible. In this case, ignorance certainly was bliss. Four toxic drugs would be involved; each had severe side-effects. Dr. Lewis called an experienced chemo nurse into the room to give us some of the details. Barry would lose his hair. There would be nausea, sores, exhaustion, and other side-effects involving the heart. This was hard to absorb. The nurse was competent and also kind. She told us as much as we could handle, and then gave us her card with an invitation to call her any time with questions. We felt that she would really be available if we needed her expertise; we were grateful. At that point, we didn't even know what to ask.

Dr. Lewis and Dr. A. were calm and reassuring. This comforted us. Dr. A. was from India, and wore a turban; Barry somehow found his sense of humor and asked if he would have to wear "one of those" when his hair fell out. We all just had to laugh at that image. How could we joke at a time like that? I guess it was our salvation. We had each other, and these competent and kind doctors to help us. I recall sitting in that exam room, numb with fear of the unknown, and watching Dr. Lewis, who was sitting on a little stool, smiling at us and chewing gum. I found that strangely reassuring; *if he could chew gum at a time like this, then how bad could it be?*

Everything seemed to happen quickly then. The chemotherapy, called MAID after the four drugs used (Mesna, Adriamycin, Ifosfamide, and DTIC), would be extremely toxic to the body. We learned that Barry could receive his treatment locally, from the oncologist who had directed us to Memorial Sloan-Kettering in the first place. He had trained at MSKCC and knew the doctors and the procedures. The recipe for the chemicals would be prescribed by Sloan, but it would be administered at the local hospital, fifteen minutes from our home. This was a tremendous relief. Within five days, my husband would have four poisonous chemo drugs coursing through his veins.

CHAPTER SIXTEEN

"MAID" CHEMOTHERAPY
(March – April '99)

The first day of chemotherapy was also the first day of Passover, a holiday we had always celebrated with a family Seder. For the past several years, it had been at our house. This year we had to skip it. One of the Seder's "Four Questions" kept echoing through my mind: *"Why is this night different from all other nights?"*

We entered the hospital at seven o'clock that first morning, since the chemo would take all day. Barry and I walked in together. He was swinging his briefcase, containing a radio and reading material. He would soon feel too ill to use any of it, but we didn't know that yet.

There were always blood tests and EKG's to be done before administering the drugs. Then we would wait for the oncologist to arrive to check the test results and give his okay to begin treatment. I remember the oncologist reading the recipe of drugs and saying, "This will be difficult." We had no idea what he meant, and that was probably a good thing. We felt that we were ready for anything. Whatever it was, we would handle it. Was there any choice?

Barry had known the head chemo nurse for many years. She had been working at the hospital when he joined the staff almost thirty years earlier. She was a big woman, kindly and competent, with a no-nonsense attitude. She herself was a survivor of two different kinds of cancer. She also had been born and raised in Arizona, so we had a lot to talk about. She was a godsend to us.

Barry was settled into the outpatient IV unit, and rested while his chemotherapy was administered. The drugs were to be given one at a time, some with specified time intervals between them. The entire routine would take until midnight. I spent the day going back and forth between the hospital and our office across the street, and doing local errands. Each time I returned to the hospital room, I found my husband more groggy, glassy-eyed, pale, and weak. The change in him was shocking.

In the afternoon, the nurses administered their last dose. Then they moved Barry in a wheel chair up to a regular hospital room, where he would stay until the final doses were finished in the evening, given by the nurses on the floor. At midnight, he was done. I wheeled Barry to the hospital door, and while an aide waited with him, I brought the car. We helped him into the car, and I drove slowly home, with my husband clutching a little pan in front of him in case he couldn't control the nausea. A perfectly strong, healthy-looking man had entered the hospital early that morning; seventeen hours later, I wheeled out a sickly, weak patient.

The following morning, the nausea was gone, and some of Barry's energy returned. When we arrived at the hospital again at 7 AM, we saw the midnight shift leaving. These were some of the same nurses who had come on duty at 11 the previous night; we had seen them come in at night, and now we waved good-bye to them as they went home in the morning. Their eyes opened in astonishment as they saw us going back into the hospital.

The chemotherapy was administered over three days, but the first day was the longest and hardest, with more drugs involved than the other two days. The first day involved the most toxic drugs, too, including the one that produced the nausea. We were never able to control that nausea, no matter what we tried.

It was sobering to see the chemo nurse pulling on heavy-duty gloves, before handling one of the drugs. This medicine was so toxic that if any of it spilled on the nurse, it would eat into her skin. The drug wouldn't damage the inside of the blood vessels, but if any of it leaked out of Barry's vein, it would be a problem. For this reason, we were continually checking to see if the IV had infiltrated. Another of the drugs was fragile and would break down if exposed to light. That medicine had to be hung on the IV pole with a brown paper bag over it, so no light touched it. Quite an operation.

The second and third days of the chemotherapy were shorter than the first, lasting only until about nine or ten in the evening. Also, the side effects of the treatments were less severe, and Barry often was able to sleep for some of the time. I spent many hours sitting in his hospital room, knitting or reading, passing the time, wondering at the situation in which we found ourselves. When I could, I went out to my karate class, returning renewed and better able to cope with it all.

We were still checking in by phone with Dr. Lewis at Sloan-Kettering, and receiving support and encouragement from him. We had no frame of reference by which to judge Barry's reactions to the chemo, and just did our best to deal with his condition day by day. But Dr. Lewis constantly reassured us that we were doing very well; this did a lot to keep our spirits up. *I wonder if people realize how much a doctor's positive attitude can do for a patient.*

The same three-day chemotherapy course was administered once a month. That meant that after these three days, we had the rest of the week to recuperate, and then had three weeks off before the next round. During the weeks off, Barry had weekly blood tests to monitor his blood counts, since low counts would make him susceptible to infection. We continued to work in between the chemo rounds, but we had to be careful of patients carrying infection into our office. Our secretaries asked every patient if he or she had a cold or flu. We were wary of going into crowds, and we watched out for people coughing or sneezing wherever we went. This became routine, and we hardly thought about it after a while. It still amazes me what we can get used to. What seems outrageous at first soon becomes routine; the human mind adapts so well.

My husband's patients were wonderful in their response to his illness. Every single one of them was supportive, many telling us that they continued to pray for him. Patients called from time to time to see how he was doing. I was surprised by this; I had felt that people would shun us or run away in fear once they knew the situation. Wrong again. The depth and beauty of the human spirit astonished me; ordinary people had so much to give.

During this time, it was essential for me to keep up the activities that renewed my sense of well-being. Karate was one of these. My classes were wonderful; I found my fellow students supportive, and I felt that I was not alone in the world. My teacher, or Sensei, was concerned about Barry and me, and I know he made allowances for my being distracted or exhausted. After class, I felt exhilarated by the strenuous physical activity (not to mention how good it was to be in a group that wasn't medical). I was able to forget everything for that brief time. As I drove home after class, alone in the darkness, I played my tape of the young guitarist we had heard in Sedona, Arizona. I was soaking wet from the exercise, the window was open with a chilly breeze blowing in my face, and the music made me cry my heart out. I didn't let out my sadness until I was alone. This was my outlet.

CHAPTER SEVENTEEN

A SUMMER OF CHEMO;
SOME GOOD LUCK
(June '99)

It was now a full year since the appearance of Barry's cancer. One year....hard to believe. We were in a new life now, the life of a cancer fighter and a caregiver. And we accepted these roles; we did whatever we had to do.

When a patient begins chemo, he and his family are given many booklets to read, containing helpful information about the treatment. You read about nausea, loss of appetite, and what the caregiver can do to help the patient maintain proper nutrition. Similar tips are given about hair loss, mouth sores and fatigue. I was determined to keep Barry in the best possible condition. I went shopping for all his favorite foods. I bought several nutritional drinks and supplements. Since he would be getting the chemo during the spring and summer, I created appetizing summertime shakes with our ancient blender, adding some of these new calcium and protein boosters. I also visited a local bakery regularly. It turned out that there was little need for all of this. Barry hardly lost his appetite. When he was nauseous, there was no question of eating, and when he felt okay, his appetite was great. But at least I felt that I was doing something to help. When he didn't experience many of the other unpleasant side effects of the medications, I attributed this to his general good health.

Something unexpected happened soon after the beginning of chemo. Since we had to wait at the hospital for several hours for the last dose of medicine to be administered, Barry and his buddy, the chemo nurse, dreamed up a scheme to allow us to go home sooner. They figured that we could leave the hospital three hours earlier if I gave Barry the last bag of IV medicine at home. The nurse would leave the IV needle in Barry's arm, and we would take the medicine home with us. When it was time to give the drugs,

I was to flush the IV, hang the bag of drugs on a curtain rod, and connect it to the IV in his arm. When I heard this, I wanted to scream! *How could they expect me to do this?* But the nurse and my husband were adamant; this would work and would be "more comfortable for everyone." I insisted that they get permission from the oncologist, which they did. *Why was this allowed?* To me, it was example of how doctors may receive worse treatment than lay patients. This would never have been suggested, had Barry not been a physician.

Once home, Barry directed me as I flushed his IV line. We hung the bag of medicine, and started the flow into his IV, but something wasn't right. Within a few seconds, Barry's arm began to swell. The IV had infiltrated his arm. We needed to stop the IV, but the drug had to be given at this precise time, since it served to counteract severe side effects of the earlier drugs. There was little leeway in the timing here. Staving off panic, we stopped the IV and I ran to the telephone, frantic. It was evening now.

First I called the home phone of the oncologist. There was no answer, so I left a message. Then I looked up the phone number of the chemo nurse in the phone book; fortunately, she was listed, and I found the number and dialed it. She was home. I apologized for the call, and told her what had happened. She told us to go right back to the hospital. She would call the second-in-command nurse in the chemo dept, who was still on duty, and would have her prepared to re-start a new IV as soon as we arrived. Barry and I jumped into our car, and I drove the ten miles back to the hospital with my heart in my throat. Within a few minutes of arriving, we were sitting in the chemo department, a new IV started, and the important drug flowing. What an experience! Needless, to say, we never tried this again!

During the second month of chemo, Barry's hair began to fall out. We had been told to expect this, but it was still very disturbing. I think this is because before this happens you still look "normal," but once your hair is gone, or is falling out, everyone who sees you knows you are on chemo. It is like wearing a sign that says "cancer patient."

Barry wanted his secretaries and me to prepare his patients for his loss of hair before they saw him. Some patients had already expressed surprise at seeing him bald. He had to explain his situation and it was uncomfortable for him. To have to say over and over that he was on chemo, and to deal with people's reactions was difficult. One elderly patient, a very tiny woman, waited until after her entire exam, and then looked up into Barry's face and said, "So, what-a happen to you hair?" We all had to laugh at this, but she sure didn't when he explained it to her. From that time on, we warned every person who went in to see Barry that he had no hair.

Now, when I say "no hair," I mean no hair anywhere: bald head, no eyebrows, no eyelashes, no hair on arms, etc. You don't realize all the places you have hair, and all the uses it serves, until you suddenly have no hair at all. Most of Barry's patients took his baldness in stride; a couple started crying; some were shocked. What I found amazing was the number who said they had been through it, or their spouses had been through it. Cancer had touched so many.

Several of our patients thought Barry looked good without hair! In fact, one dignified older patient, who was outspoken, to put it mildly, thought Barry looked better bald than with hair. From the first day she saw him bald she insisted that he looked better than he ever had, and when she saw him months later, after his hair had started to grow back, she told me to make him shave his head! People are funny. Though this experience is behind me, something remains. Whenever I see a bald head, the first thing I do is look for the person's eyebrows. If I see them, I know the person has shaved his head as a fashion statement; if there are no eyebrows, I think, *this person is on chemo.*

After the first two months of chemo, Barry was to have a CAT scan to see if the drugs were having an effect. Then there would be a pause in the chemo, during which chest surgery was planned. The thoracic surgeon at Memorial Sloan-Kettering would remove as much of the "tumor load" as he could, and, after some recuperation, chemo would resume for four more months.

The CAT scan was scheduled at our local hospital on a Wednesday, and we waited anxiously at our office to hear from the radiologist. He called not long after with the results: the lungs were clear! Every one of the lung lesions had disappeared! This was a greater response than anyone had dared to hope for. To us it was unbelievable. We were in shock, but this was "good" shock. My emotions went from intense fear to relief in a few minutes. Yes, we were very lucky. As Dr. Lewis explained later to us, the tumor's response to the chemo was a function of its biology: apparently, it was susceptible to this combination of drugs. This was something that nobody could anticipate; you just had to administer the chemo and wait to see how the tumor responded.

What to do now? Why have major chest surgery on both lungs if the tumors were gone? We met with the chest surgeon, Dr. A., at Sloan-Kettering, and he told us that the surgery would not be necessary. We were thrilled. This was surely a miracle. We had hope and a future again!

We still had to complete the course of chemo. But it is a very different matter to have chemo that you know is working, than it is to undergo it when you don't know if it is doing anything. The next four months were spent in the difficult chemo-regime, but with a hopeful attitude.

Not all of the side effects of the chemotherapy made Barry feel sick. One of the drugs given with the chemo was a steroid that tended to make patients "hyper." After certain days of the treatment, my husband simply could not sit still. I might be mentally and physically drained by our ordeal, but Barry was "revved up." If we stopped at our office as we did sometimes on the day after the chemo, Barry would start rearranging things, cleaning and making repairs. At home, he became Mr. Fix-it. He cleaned, shined, repaired, rejuvenated, and repainted everything he could reach. When the effects of the medication wore off, he crashed, but the routine was predictable and we found it funny. I would be lying down, exhausted, while my husband, the patient, was painting our front door, or something like that.

One summer evening during chemo, when Barry was in the hospital room getting the last dose of his medicine, I kept encountering a young woman in the hallway. She looked familiar, but I couldn't recall how I knew her. When she said hello to me for the umpteenth time, I finally asked her who she was. "I'm your lifeguard!" she replied with a grin. Of course, of course! (I hadn't recognized her without her bathing suit.) It was common for us swimmers, if we met each other in town, to say, "Oh, hi, I didn't recognize you with your clothes on!" We thought we were so funny. Our lifeguard was spending evenings in the hospital with her mother, who had brain cancer. The outlook was not good, and this young college student had become the caregiver for her mother. Here was a young, valiant person dealing with another one of life's nasty surprises.

Barry and I took several mini-vacations that summer, sandwiched between chemo treatments. We drove to Ithaca, our old favorite spot in upstate New York. We relaxed along the shores of Lake Cayuga, and strolled through the gorges outside of town. Ithaca is filled with old Victorian homes on streets lined with ancient shade trees. It is like a town back in the nineteenth century. When it gets too hot in town, you can always cool off in one of the deep gorges, or catch the breeze coming off the lake. For us, remembering our college days there, it was a great vacation spot.

Hurricane Floyd hit New York in September, right in the middle of a chemo week. It arrived in the evening on the second day of Barry's three-day treatment. We were at the hospital and Barry was having his last dose of the day. Outside the wind was raging. Rain pelted the hospital windows. It was dark, and the lights in the hospital parking lot showed the rain blowing sideways. Waves of water rushed along the street. We had to get home through this, and return early the next morning. Some of the nurses who had long distances to travel home were staying overnight at the hospital. That's what I wanted to do. Even if we made it home safely, how would we get back the next morning? I wondered whether the roads would be clear, since trees were sure to come down in this storm. But my husband was adamant: he wanted to go home and to sleep in his own bed. Only his own bed seemed comforting and he didn't want to stay in the hospital and feel like a patient any longer than he had to. I was now the caregiver, the driver, the protector. So I put our Jeep in four-wheel drive, and said a little prayer. With all the skill I could muster, I ferried us the ten miles home through deep water and ferocious winds, trying my best to stay away from the other unfortunate souls out on the roads on a night like that. Somehow we made it home, slowly but surely, and even made it back for our usual seven 7 o'clock treatment the next morning.

Another big event for us that summer was my karate test for Second Degree Black Belt, or Nidan. I had continued karate classes whenever I could throughout Barry's illness. I really had to concentrate in class, and it took my mind off everything else. Barry recognized this, and was happy to see me leave for class, knowing I would return refreshed and rejuvenated. He didn't want to see me worn down by his disease. As the day neared for my big test, I got nervous, of course, but I was excited. I felt prepared. Barry came to videotape the test. He always did that, and feeling weak or being bald was not going to stop him now. I was proud of both of us that night.

Near the end of the summer, we took another long weekend trip to Rockport and Gloucester, Mass. Barry and I had lived in Boston when we were first married, during his surgical internship, and we had explored Cape Ann at that time. It had been a quick getaway from his duties in medical training, and it provided a change of pace for us now as well. Cape Ann is similar to Cape Cod, jutting out into the Atlantic, a little north of Boston, and its towns have the flavor of small, New England fishing villages. Places with names like Annisquam, Good Harbor Beach, Folly Cove, and Bearskin Neck conjure up times past. We have been there in all seasons, and find it glorious with its many sailboats and fishing boats. You can walk all day along the beaches, or on the winding village streets, or just laze in the shade. It did wonders for us: it made us feel normal again. And we were coming to the end of chemo!

At home, when we wanted a change of scenery, we would drive over to the park along the Hudson River, the one we had found the previous year, during the radiation treatment. It was a beautiful spot, and transported us to entirely new surroundings without going far. We could stroll along the paths, or take a long hike, if we had the energy. On one of these outings, I suggested that we stop in at the radiation facility and say hello. I knew that the nurses and technicians would be curious about how Barry was doing. The last time we had communicated, it was to cancel our last check-up there, because of the return of the sarcoma and the subsequent chemo regimen. There was little follow-up information for these dedicated young people, who saw patients intensely during their radiation, but then never knew what happened to them afterwards. So we went to our old haunt, the radiation building, and were proud to show several of the technicians and nurses how well Barry looked. The staff was delighted to see him. I wanted to ask about the young girl whose last day had coincided with our first day there, the one whose sarcoma had been even larger than my husband's. We dreaded hearing about her, fearing the worst. But I found the courage to ask, and there was good news: she was fine! This made us feel great. Another success story; another miracle.

CHAPTER EIGHTEEN

LIFE AFTER CHEMO
(Oct '99)

Chemotherapy ended on September 17, 1999. Six weeks later we were in Arizona. This was "doctor's orders," and we didn't need much coaxing. We could hardly believe that the chemo was over; it had been six months of poison, sickness, weakness, and fear, yet it had saved Barry's life. Again I felt so grateful to the doctors, nurses, and researchers whose dedication had enabled us to have the medical treatment we needed. Now Barry's CAT scans showed clear lungs. He would live.

We were so used to medical procedures, IV's, and hospital rooms that it seemed weird to be released from all of that. The normal seemed foreign, and the strange had become familiar. But now we were on vacation, just like all the other people at the Grand Canyon. We didn't have to worry about cancer; all we had to do was heal. Arizona was a wonderful place to do it.

We enjoyed all of our usual spots in northern Arizona, but slowly, all the while, pinching ourselves to be sure that we were really there. It was a week of relaxation, and of relishing the glorious scenery in that part of the state. And also of thanking our lucky stars that we had lived through the past six months and had the good fortune to be able to enjoy ourselves out west again. We sat once more in the sun at Tlaquepaque, listening to our wonderful guitar player. So much had changed in our lives in one year, and yet, that young man stood there in the same spot, playing his songs and smiling, just as before.

When we returned from vacation it was November, and we became busy with work and plans for the holidays. We had family parties to give, a play of our daughter's to see in the city, walks and dinners with friends, and time to just enjoy being alive. The time between vacation and the end of the year went by, and we were still finding it hard to grasp all we had been through, and that it was finally over. On New Year's Eve, we celebrated the millennium with everyone else on the planet, but we were really celebrating much, much more.

With the new year, we were determined to have a more normal life. We decided to plan our annual trip to the West for February, and also to re-plan the visit to Sara and Richard in Alaska for the following June. This was the trip we had cancelled the previous year due to Barry's recurrence and the summer of chemo. There were lots of details to work out for this trip, so I concentrated on it and got it done as quickly as possible. It was fun talking to the Alaska State Ferry office on the telephone, and making the plans for all the towns we wanted to visit.

We had a January CAT scan to get through before we went on vacation. The CAT scan showed clean lungs again; we began to relax a little. I realized that a good strategy would be to plan any trips we wanted to make for the periods just before any scheduled scans. That way, whatever the x-rays showed, we would have already had our vacation, and there would be no plans to cancel. I was adapting to our situation.

All this time we had continued to talk to Dr. Lewis from Sloan-Kettering weekly. We had become real friends. Barry often said that this wonderful man was like a brother to him. I still cannot understand how such a busy man found the time to give us such support. *Did he do this with everybody?* One time we were discussing the nervous tension that preceded every CAT scan, and Dr. Lewis asked us if it would help us if he or his office called us the day before each scan. We said no, but were amazed at the offer. He told us about another patient, a man who got so nervous before each scan that his wife would schedule the tests without telling him; then, the day of the scan, she would tell him that they were going to the hospital. That way, he didn't have the anxiety of anticipation.

I was aware of how much Dr. Lewis was involved with at work, and it is still a mystery to me how this busy man was able to be so giving. I often wondered if he were more than human. I am not a religious person, but this was almost enough to make me one. I fantasized that, years in the future, we would stop in at Memorial Sloan-Kettering Cancer Center, and ask to say hello to Dr. Lewis, and someone would say to us, "Dr. Who? No, we never had a Dr. Lewis here." Then we would know that, indeed, he had been our guardian angel.

CHAPTER NINETEEN

"NORMALITY" – ADJUSTMENTS
(Feb – March '00)

Life returned to normal, and normal was heavenly. We had thought we would never feel normal again, yet here we were, doing routine things and feeling relaxed without looking over our shoulders every minute. We knew that this could change at any moment. The next CAT scan could bring us to our knees, and this was part of what made life so precious and so beautiful. It's too bad people can't appreciate things this way without the experience of a life-threatening illness.

We noticed a strange phenomenon throughout our treatment experience: as soon as a certain treatment was over, our minds blocked it out. We forgot it. It was almost if the treatment never happened. What I mean is that we did not dwell on what had just happened; we focused on the next stage of our life. If things seemed fine, we didn't think about the treatment at all. When something happened that jogged our memories, we remembered everything including every tiny detail, but even these memories didn't linger in our consciousness. I think it's a "survival thing" to look forward, not back. Sometimes Barry would remark that he could hardly believe that all this was happening to him. It was as if he were watching a movie about someone else. I knew what he meant; I felt the same way.

We made our February visit to the southwest and it was just what we needed to forget the past year. The chemo year. But it was over now, and now we were in Arizona. We spent the first weekend driving to California, as we had the previous year, to visit my aunt, uncle, cousins, and their children. It was like old times.

We took a new route through the high desert back to Arizona, stopping overnight in Prescott. It's an old, old town with authentic western flavor, although lately it has been attracting many new residents.

From Prescott we wound our way up over Mingus Mountain, through the little ghost town of Jerome, and north to Sedona and Flagstaff. As always, we found a few clear days to run up to the Grand Canyon, delighting in our usual views of it with its winter blanket. While in the north country, we had some days of drizzle and fog. You would look down into the Canyon at the breathtaking view, and in front of your eyes the Canyon walls would disappear as clouds dropped down and filled the abyss. You knew that the cavern lay in front of you, but could see nothing but white mist.

Back at home, Barry tried to fit into his old life. It was not easy. Did he really want to work as hard as he had before? Physically, it was difficult, if not impossible. For one thing, surgery was out. It had been a long time since he had performed operations, actually since just before his own surgery at Sloan a year and a half ago. Surgery had been such a big part of Barry's identity in prior years that I wondered how he could give it up. But he could. It helped that several other doctors around his age were also giving up surgery or thinking about retiring. Life was changing, and not only because of his illness. And the cancer, and chance of recurrence, weighed on his mind. Barry felt that if he had only months or a year to live, he didn't want to spend the time working. On the other hand, if he had years left, then why retire right now? We decided not to make any big decisions just yet. We would take it slow and see how things played out.

We developed a schedule: after an early swim, we worked mornings in the office and took most afternoons off. Occasionally, we scheduled an afternoon of appointments for patients who needed them. It was almost like semi-retirement. But we needed afternoons for paperwork, errands, and for Barry's medical care. He found it difficult to stand all day in the office anyway, since his leg had not been the same after the removal of so much muscle, vein, and nerve. And we still needed time for his CAT scans and check-ups at Sloan-Kettering.

This schedule gave us many afternoons to "smell the roses." We eased back into life. We were becoming accustomed to enjoying the beauty around us, and taking the time every day to listen to music and appreciate nature. We walked in the Rockefeller park along the Hudson River, high above its busy waters. We tried to imagine the

way it had looked a hundred years before, without the traffic or the
Tappan Zee Bridge, or the highways along the shores of the river.
We discovered a beach and nature preserve in Connecticut open to
the public December through March, and enjoyed walking along the
water. It was just across Long Island Sound from Huntington, where
I had grown up. We found many unusual birds there, some nesting,
and we could see New York City from the beach. I often gazed out
across the water at the Twin Towers of the World Trade Center, and
thought about our daughter Ellen working just a few blocks from
there.

On our quiet afternoons, we learned to take naps when our
bodies told us to. We were older, and had just survived nearly two
hellish years. We needed to slow down a little, to renew ourselves. I
was able to take more time to pursue my art. After years of painting,
I was now an art-quilter, and appreciated time to concentrate more
fully on my work. Barry and I were making adjustments, and we
didn't see any point in rushing through life as we had in the past.
It was more important to take our time, and to live fully every day,
paying attention to each moment. I recognized the wonderful family
we had: our two children, our son-in-law, my mother, my brother and
his family, and our various aunts, uncles and cousins, not to mention
old and new friends who had been so supportive, and our kind Dr.
Lewis. They were all special to us, and we didn't feel alone in the
world. Barry and I felt so lucky to have each other, something that
we no longer took for granted. We had met when we were both very
young, and now we appreciated the specialness of being together for
so many years. Whatever differences of opinion we had, even some
that had loomed large before, seemed insignificant now. We were
united in fighting a common enemy.

Our next CAT scan was in April. This time, the scan showed a
small spot on Barry's liver. The radiologists at our local hospital and
at Sloan-Kettering read it as a hemangioma, something similar to a
birthmark. That was good enough for us; we weren't looking for any
trouble, and we didn't want to be second-guessing the specialists.
We told ourselves, *if they said it was a hemangioma, then it must be.*
If we were worried, we buried the feelings until the next scan.

We had regular appointments every three months with Dr. Lewis at Sloan-Kettering. He was always encouraging. During one of our visits, I asked him about a lump on Barry's leg where the original tumor had been. After the surgery, fluid had collected there, and, as Dr. Lewis had predicted, it had not gone away or reabsorbed. It was not a medical problem, but it didn't look normal, and I was wondering whether it would ever go away, or whether they could do anything about it. Dr. Lewis said that if they did try to remove it, more fluid would probably collect there as a result of the anatomy changes after the surgery. He said with his characteristic smile, "That's your lucky bump!"

On the train ride home from New York City after an appointment at Sloan, we bumped into our chemo nurse from the previous year before. We had promised to keep in touch with each other, especially since she had retired just as Barry was finishing his chemo, but naturally we all had gotten busy with the details of life. It was great to see her; she looked relaxed and happy. But since she, too, was a cancer survivor, she had to have regular check-ups and tests. At that time she also had something suspicious that was being watched by her doctors. The three of us were like people bobbing in a life raft in the middle of the ocean.

So the spring was spent readjusting to life; seeing another new play Ellen was directing, feeding the neighbors' cat, getting the lawn mowed as in other years. In May, we went to visit a young cousin of my husband's who had a brain tumor and had come to New York to visit family. Relatives thought that Barry could encourage this young man to go ahead with treatment, rather than give up, as he was inclined to do. He was in dire straits; he had had radiation to the brain, and had damage related to that. His speech was slurred, he walked haltingly, much of his hair was missing, and I'm sure there were other effects which were less obvious to us. He was discouraged. He wanted to stop treatment and to be left to die in peace.

We wanted to help in any way we could, and talking to Barry might be just what this young man needed. They took a walk together, and Barry told him about his own experiences with chemo, surgery, radiation, and the fantastic doctors at Sloan-Kettering. Later, I added my encouragement. We were enthusiastic about trying every option available, and he could see how well Barry looked and felt, which was amazing after so much cancer treatment. He could see that there was hope for cancer patients. We left that visit feeling that we had been able to give back a portion of the care that had been given to us. Somehow, I realized that my belief in fighting for your life had grown stronger and stronger, possibly because of all the courageous people we met.

CHAPTER TWENTY

ALASKA OR BUST!
(June '00)

Finally it was June, two years into our cancer life, and time for our long-postponed trip to Alaska! I had carefully planned each detail, and could hardly wait to see that beautiful state, and to give my daughter and son-in-law a big hug! You become very clever about life with cancer, and we had scheduled the trip just prior our next CAT scan so that nothing could interfere with our vacation.

Our flight took us to Anchorage, and as we landed, the snow-covered mountains surrounding the city took our breath away. We relaxed and explored some of the town before heading north to Fairbanks where Sara and Richard lived. Anchorage was unlike anything we had ever seen. We were struck by the rugged mountains that provided the backdrop for the city. It felt like a frontier town: raw, wild, on the edge of wilderness. And this was the largest city in the state...

Driving north, we stopped for the night at Denali Park. We had been told we might not be able to see Mt. McKinley as it is often shrouded in fog or clouds. But as we drove, we had clear views of the mountain, snow-covered and massive. I had never had the wish to be a mountain climber, but McKinley had a magnetism that made me want to get close to it.

The following morning, we continued north to Fairbanks, stopping briefly at a little town called Nenana to see the famous Alaskan Railroad. Nenana consisted of the railroad station, a bar, and a few houses: a relic of Alaska's frontier days. We drove on to Fairbanks, where we met Sara and Richard at a bagel shop on the outskirts of town for brunch. They wanted to lead us to their house, knowing that we might have trouble finding it on our own. They were right.

They lived on Grubstake Road, a dirt road off another dirt road, up high on the northeast side of town, with views of mountains and the valley for miles around. Their house was tiny and adorable and we learned that they had spent the previous four days feverishly painting the inside! It looked great, and we were touched by their efforts. We had sent them several decorative wall hangings from our own house, and it was strange to see these familiar things in an Alaskan wilderness setting. We were seeing the next generation starting out in married life, when we didn't yet feel old enough to be the "older generation" ourselves.

The week we spent in Fairbanks was wonderful. Barry and I expected to give Sara and Richard some time to themselves, but all of us wanted to spend as much time together as possible. We didn't know when we would see each other again. So we saw the sights around Fairbanks, and Sara and Richard drove us out of town to their favorite spots. We saw the end of paved road in North America, where a dirt and gravel road continued on to Barrow. We visited an old gold mine north of town, and ate lunch in a typical Alaskan cafe, complete with antlers mounted over the door. We discovered that many of the buildings had antlers over the doors, and that many of the houses were log cabins. We went to a park with a man-made lake east of town, where a dam had been built to prevent the two rivers that flowed through town from flooding it, a frequent problem in the past. And, of course, we saw the old ferryboat, a "sternwheeler," which takes tourists up and down the river, repeating the trips of a hundred years ago.

We took many photographs and videos, and spent hours walking or just being together. But we couldn't stop the time from running out. We left Fairbanks for several days of travel on our own, before meeting Sara and Richard again at Kenai Fjords National Park. Barry and I drove south towards Prince William Sound, heading for Valdez, marveling at the scenery every inch of the way. I kept a sharp eye out for wildlife, and we were rewarded with glimpses of bear, porcupine, moose, and Dall sheep on the mountainsides.

Barry looked and felt fantastic. We were able to put our worries about his medical condition in the back of our minds. But when we browsed through the local gift shops, he wouldn't buy even a shirt for himself unless I promised to give it to our son-in-law if "something happened." Somehow, in this complex frame of mind, we pressed on, able to give ourselves fully to this exciting adventure.

Valdez was a small, beautiful town, built on the edge of Prince William Sound, with magnificent mountains that rose up behind it. The weather was misty and rainy, but that only added to the atmosphere. We marveled that people lived in such an isolated spot on this small strip of land on the edge of the water. From Valdez, we boarded the Alaska State Ferry with our rented car, and sailed across the choppy water to Whittier, a village so small that you could hardly call it a settlement. The only thing we could see was the ferry terminal, along with a few lodgings for the handful of people who worked in it. We drove on to Seward, where we would stay for several days.

Seward was a place we could really enjoy. The scenery was beyond anything we could have imagined, with snow-covered mountains looming in every direction, and the port on Resurrection Bay dominating the town. It was a base for fishing boats, and for tour boats that carried visitors into Kenai Fjords National Park. We had reserved one of these tours for ourselves and Sara and Richard. A few days after we arrived in Seward, they joined us, after making the twelve hour drive down from Fairbanks.

It had been drizzling and misty every day since we arrived in Seward, but on the day of our boat trip the sun shone bright and early. Even with calm seas and sunshine, the trip was rough, and all of us except our hardy son-in-law fought off seasickness. Still, the boat ride was a highlight of our vacation because of the wildlife we saw and because of the beauty of the shoreline. We spent the entire day aboard, and delighted in the breaching whales, puffins, sea lions, eagles, sea otters, and kittiwakes along the way. We also saw glaciers "calving," and spent an hour just bobbing up and down amid icebergs, waiting for the blue ice of the glacier to fall thunderously into the bay. For this June trip we had been advised to dress in winter coats, with hats, scarves and gloves. We needed it all.

After the boat trip, we took an emotional leave of our daughter and son-in-law. Do you know how hard it is to leave your daughter?

The only thing that kept me from becoming despondent was that she and Richard looked so happy. How many times did I tell myself that? Did I want her living down the street from me, when her heart was full of adventure? Well….. We continued our travels, as they headed home. Our last stop was Homer, a little town at the end of the Kenai Peninsula. Barry's radiation nurse had recommended this spot, and we didn't want to miss it. The drive there circled the entire peninsula, with westward views of the Aleutian Islands with their volcanic peaks. Homer was a tiny town, with few places for tourists to stay, or even to eat. It had the atmosphere of a working fishing village. Many vacationers had come here to fish as well. You could see the boats heading from Katchemack Bay out to sea very early in the morning, returning with their catch each afternoon, and laying the huge fish out on the docks.

After a day and night in Homer, we had to head back to Anchorage to catch our plane home. What a wonderful trip we had had, and how good it was to be alive!

CHAPTER TWENTY-ONE

BACK HOME
(July '00)

Within two weeks of returning home, Barry was lying on the CAT scan table again, with the "rays of truth" coursing through him. When the radiologists at Sloan-Kettering read the films this time, they couldn't agree on what they saw. One specialist thought the small mass on his liver was a hemangioma, while the other read it as a metastasis of the original sarcoma tumor. We met with Dr. Lewis to discuss our options. The doctor could biopsy the mass, but it was close to the lung and there was a risk of a puncture. An alternate was to wait a month and to repeat the scan to see whether the spot had changed. We decided to wait the month, as long as we were not jeopardizing Barry by waiting.

But now there was another wrinkle: our compassionate Dr. Lewis, who had guided us through the trials of the past two and a half years, would be leaving his medical practice at Memorial Sloan-Kettering Cancer Center. What on earth would we do without him? Dr. Lewis had intimated that he was reviewing his work options a few months earlier. He had decided to shift his focus entirely to pure research, and would not be providing patient care after August, which was about a month away. Still, he assured us that he would continue to take care of us, and we had faith that he would do what he promised.

We were anxious during the month leading to the next scan. It helped us to get away for a week-end in upstate New York again. We had both been to college in Ithaca, and although Barry's last year had coincided with my first year, we hadn't met then. We met the following summer, when we both were camp counselors. Our summer romance lingered into the fall, when Barry started medical school and I returned to college. During that school year, we visited each other almost every week-end, which wasn't good for our studies. Nevertheless, time after time, Barry drove his old Ford through snow and ice to visit me upstate. How many times did that car break down en route, or in sub-zero Ithaca? How many times did I hold the flashlight for him as he tried to fix something under the car? I recall one evening, when Barry was driving me back to my dormitory. We encountered a ferocious fire in downtown Ithaca, with flames shooting skyward out of the old, wooden buildings. Fire trucks were lined up on the main street, firemen standing high up in raised buckets shooting water onto the blaze, but as soon as the water hit the buildings, it froze. Huge icicles hung down, almost to the ground. It was mesmerizing, but we had to tear ourselves away to get me back to my dorm by curfew.

Curfew: what an outdated concept. At Cornell, girls had to sign out in order to leave the dorm in the evening, and sign back in before the 10 PM deadline. Monitors sat at the front desk of the dorm to enforce these rules. After all, in those days, the college was operating "in loco parentis." Women's liberation and coed dorms hadn't been heard of then.

These early memories of Cornell were etched into our minds, and a visit to Ithaca brought them vividly back; it was such a pleasure to vacation there. It was one place that could distract us from our present-day worries.

When we returned home, Barry repeated the CAT scan. We Fed-Exed the films to the radiologist at Sloan-Kettering. This time the specialists speculated that Barry had a metastasized sarcoma tumor in his liver.

We met with Dr. Lewis on what was to be his last day of practice at Sloan-Kettering, and told us he would set up a meeting for us a few days later with a Sloan oncologist. Before we left the office that day, Barry shocked me when he turned to Dr. Lewis somberly and asked, "Will you help me die?" I held my breath and tried to appear calm, but inside my stomach was churning and my head throbbed. I tried to blot this all out of my mind. *It couldn't be happening.* I knew that Barry was afraid of dying in pain, without sufficient medication, and he trusted Dr. Lewis to be compassionate. Our caring doctor simply replied, "I will not abandon you." How difficult that must have been for him.

Three days later we met the oncologist. His lack of evident compassion caused us a fair amount of anxiety despite his intelligence and expertise. I guess that this must have been his way of coping with so much sadness and tragedy. I was so distressed when we left his office that I could not find my way from the exam room to the waiting room. I have an excellent sense of direction; I never get lost; yet I could not retrace my steps down a hallway and through the door marked "Exit." The destructive power of anxiety cannot be overestimated.

Having survived the appointment, we arranged for the two months of chemotherapy he suggested, which again could be administered at our local hospital by the oncologist we had known for years. We still had support from Dr. Lewis, who checked in with us frequently to be sure we were doing all right. He knew we would need encouragement after our difficult visits with the oncologist.

Barry still looked and felt great; it was hard to believe that something malignant was growing inside of him. He was active, still working, still swimming, and enjoying puttering around the house, making improvements and keeping things in good repair. He climbed up onto the roof in the summertime to check things out. I knew that when he felt strong, he would get out the ladder from time to time and climb up and look around. This told me he felt good. I was surprised that his leg was strong enough for him to climb a tall ladder and maneuver himself onto the peaked roof. Several times, in an effort to let Dr. Lewis know how good Barry was feeling, I told him that Barry felt "good enough to climb up onto the roof." Apparently, Dr. Lewis didn't understand wanting to do this sort of thing, because one day he said to me, with bewilderment, "What does he do up there?" It must have sounded comical to him to hear me say repeatedly that Barry was up on the roof. Either you like to climb up on your roof, or you don't.

The new chemo was given once a week, and had minimal side-effects. Barry could still work, and do most other things. In the midst of all this, one of our office secretaries told us she was leaving; she was retiring and moving to New England. She had been with us for many years, and we were extremely fond of one another. In fact, she had delayed her retirement for at least a year (to the dismay of her husband) in order to be with us while Barry was going through his treatment. Now her husband was insistent, and she had to do what was right for her family. So we started putting ads in the local papers and interviewing new secretaries in between chemo doses. What a time!

CHAPTER TWENTY-TWO

AUTUMN
(Oct '00)

As luck would have it, we managed to find a new secretary for our office, and to complete the chemo, all in October. We also reached our thirty-fifth wedding anniversary, one which I know Barry thought he would never see. We had already bought ourselves a present. We had seen a lovely bowl in a local store that carried art items made in New Zealand. The bowl was crafted from rich, red jarrah wood, and from a fossilized stone that looked like green and white marble. The artist had joined these two very different materials together in graceful curves. We never bought things like this, but the bowl caught our eye, and we kept coming back to it in the store. This was an unusual purchase for us, especially with looming medical bills, but when Barry wanted it so much, I agreed to get it because this told me he believed he had a future. So we bought it for each other for our anniversary. When I looked at it in profile across our living room, it looked like a "victory bowl." It gave me hope.

I had learned that to make it through cancer treatment, we needed to give ourselves treats. This, along with physical exercise, helped us maintain a positive attitude. To that end, I planned our long weekend away for the period between the end of chemo and the next scans. We had just one weekend free, and we decided to drive down to Gettysburg, Pa. My brother and his wife would drive up from their home in Virginia and meet us there. The four of us could have a relaxing weekend, and enjoy sightseeing and dinners together. This mini-vacation was just what we needed. In the mornings, Barry and I usually were up and about long before Bruce and Jane. This gave us time to eat something at the motel's breakfast bar, take a walk together, and return to the hotel for a second cup of coffee. By this time my brother and his wife would be eating breakfast. This worked for all of us: we could have our differences and still enjoy our time together.

The October MRI and CAT scan proved problematic. The mass in Barry's liver was still there, and after two months of chemo, it had grown slightly. Nobody knew what to make of this. The experts had been looking at this spot for six months now and still couldn't tell what it was for sure. But there was one more test we had not yet had - a PET scan, and the doctors decided to try it. This was the newest type of scan. It was designed to detect cancer anywhere in the body by measuring how fast cells were multiplying.

We traveled down to New York City for the PET scan, hopeful despite our fears. Dr. Lewis had been encouraging; the mass had not grown by much, and Barry still looked and felt great. *How could this be a recurrence?* The PET scan went well, and we returned home to await the report. Two days later we had another appointment with the Sloan-Kettering oncologist, Dr. K. The PET scan showed no cancer at all, but Dr. K. was not convinced. *How was he able to so totally discount this scan?* He said he would consider this mass malignant until proven otherwise; he had his "own reasons" for not being convinced by the PET scan. He offered us an array of chemo drugs to try, none very promising, he said. The alternative was to wait for two months and to repeat a CAT scan. We asked him what he would recommend. He said it wouldn't be a bad idea to take two months off. Two months off. It didn't sound like, "You might be okay." It sounded like a break and then more treatment of some sort. But we didn't listen to the details or the innuendos. We took the two months off. Then we would face the future. We had already lived through two and a half years with cancer; we could deal with it.

CHAPTER TWENTY-THREE

SURPRISE FAMILY VACATION
(Dec '00)

It was late fall, and winter was approaching when we had our two-month respite from treatment. I decided to take the bull by the horns, be positive, and book a trip to our beloved Arizona. We could really relax there. The scenery would be good for our souls. And our annual February trip there seemed unlikely: the next few months were a big question mark for us.

I was on the telephone with Sara, telling her about our plans for Arizona, when she said to me, "Gee, I wish I could join you there." That was my wish, too. Barry and I had been hoping that she and her husband would come home for the holiday season this year. But now that they owned a home in Alaska, they were afraid to leave it in the dead of winter: any problem with the heating system or the power would mean a great loss to them. This meant that we didn't know when we would see her next. A plan was hatching in my mind. Maybe she could meet us in Arizona for a short visit. What a surprise that would be for Barry!

I suggested she call Ellen in Manhattan to see if the two of them could get away at the same time and meet us in Arizona. She loved the idea. Within days, a plan was taking shape. Sara and Ellen would fly to Phoenix, one from New York and one from Fairbanks, and meet each other the night before Barry and I arrived. They would take a shuttle north to Sedona, where we always stayed. The next day, when Barry and I arrived, our daughters would surprise us at the hotel. Brilliant!

I was so excited about this trip that I sometimes forgot my worry about Barry's condition. He was still feeling good, and I was having a good time planning our surprise. The trip would also be an early birthday present, since Barry's 60th birthday was coming up in January.

The planning involved many secret phone calls to hotels in Arizona, to the shuttle company, and to our daughters. Our emails to each other had to be concealed so Barry would not discover our plan. I was enjoying this, and in my excitement I had to be careful about not spilling the beans. I didn't even tell my mother or my brother, in case they might let something slip out. Instead, I wrote them notes, along with our itinerary which I sent them just before a trip. I mailed the letters to arrive the day we left. All went off perfectly; I don't know how.

On our flight to Phoenix I could barely contain my excitement. We landed, picked up a rental car and headed north. I knew Sara and Ellen were up in Sedona already, enjoying the day together in a town where we had spent many family vacations when they were children. Now they would see it in a new light, as adults. And I was happy that they had time alone together.

As Barry drove us north from Phoenix clouds swirled above us, dark with brilliant sunny highlights. At one point, the road curved down a steep hill, and we could see the red rocks of Sedona off towards the northwest. As we caught a glimpse of them, a rainbow appeared, ending exactly where I knew our daughters were waiting. Suddenly, it became a double rainbow! I was speechless.

We turned into the motel driveway, and I jumped out of the car, saying that I would get the key to our room. I didn't want Barry to come into the office with me, in case the clerk might say that our daughters had arrived already. As we walked to our room, we saw part of a face peering out of a neighboring room, but Barry didn't recognize it; he thought it was a child peeking out of the curtains. No sooner had we closed the motel door than there was a knock. A voice said, "Room service!" I stepped back so that Barry could be closer to the door than I was. He looked at me with wonderment: we hadn't ordered room service - this motel didn't even have room service. I motioned for him to answer the door. I wish I could have photographed the look on his face when he opened the door. There were our two daughters. Barry was flabbergasted. He had never guessed our secret. He said later that this was the best gift anyone could have given him.

The four of us spent a fabulous four days in Sedona and Flagstaff. We knew the area so well, and Sara and Ellen remembered much of it from years ago. Best of all, Barry and I took them on several of our favorite hikes. They were astounded by the natural beauty. You really can't remember the magnificence of it. Every time we have been there, we say we will hold onto it, but you just can't. As we drove down through Oak Creek Canyon one afternoon, I turned to find our younger daughter, Sara, crying. "I forgot how beautiful it is," she said.

An unexpected highlight of the vacation for me was a biplane ride over Sedona. I had looked at the tourist biplane rides at the Sedona airport for years, teasing Barry about going on one. But I wasn't serious, since my husband suffered from air-sickness. Now our daughter Ellen was fascinated, and I could see that she really wanted to try it. When she said that she thought she would like a ride, I thought it over for about a minute and said I would join her. We did it! The day was calm and gorgeous, and while Barry and Sara (who also tended to air-sickness) watched, Ellen and I went sailing off into the blue. The plane was a bright red, open-cockpit biplane, and, to put it mildly, I was terrified! But it was exhilarating. At the end of the flight, customers get a videotape that shows the aerial view of the red rocks, but also a view of the passengers themselves, complete with facial expressions. What a souvenir!

Before we knew it, our daughters had to return to their busy lives, and Barry and I were alone for the rest of our week's vacation. We managed to take an overnight run up to the Grand Canyon, and the snow on the canyon's formations was magnificent. When the trip was behind us, we were left with the most wonderful memories we have ever had. What could be better than spending time with your family in your favorite spot on earth? Especially when we didn't expect Barry to still be alive. We didn't know it then, but this was to be Barry's last visit to Arizona.

CHAPTER TWENTY-FOUR

THE TRUTH
(Dec '00 – Jan '01)

Back in New York during the holidays, we enjoyed family and friends while preparing ourselves for the CAT scan in January. We hadn't seen Dr. Lewis in about six months, but he had continued to follow Barry's condition closely. His schedule was hectic now, filled with traveling, but he still managed to take care of us. Since Dr. Lewis hadn't seen my husband in a while, he could evaluate Barry's condition just by observing how his appearance had changed. Dr. Lewis encouraged us, saying that Barry wouldn't look or feel this well if something terrible were going on. His optimism was such a help to us during periods of uncertainty or stress; he exuded a feeling of confidence, of being able to deal with whatever turned up. Dr. Lewis's encouragement enabled us to go on without sinking into depression. His positive outlook was something that I tried consciously to adopt.

Soon it was January, and time for the dreaded CAT scan. Again, the findings were unclear. The specialists still couldn't tell whether the mass was cancer or a benign lesion. There was only one thing left to do, and there was no postponing it now. We would have to have a needle biopsy performed by an interventional radiologist at Sloan-Kettering. We had tried to avoid this because there were serious risks involved. The needle might puncture the lungs, causing a pneumothorax, which would involve putting a chest tube in. And if the lesion were a hemangioma, uncontrolled bleeding might occur. We had been hoping that one of the various scans would tell us the answer without our having to take this step, but it hadn't. Now there was no way around it; we simply had to find out what was growing on Barry's liver.

We drove to Manhattan very early on the morning of the biopsy. The sun was rising over the skyline as we neared the city. It was a glorious sight. There was not much traffic, and we sailed along in our Jeep, with the sunrise blazing in the east, a breathtaking moon lingering low in the western sky.

The procedure went smoothly. The radiologist was competent and reassuring, and none of our fears materialized. The only hitch was that Barry's blood pressure dropped precipitously a little while after the procedure, but he was resting in the recovery room at the time, so all the medical personnel he needed were right there. Before we knew it, we were on our way home, and the whole process was over. We didn't expect to hear the results until the following week, when we were scheduled to meet with our dour Sloan-Kettering oncologist.

We resumed work at Barry's office, and the day after the biopsy, when we returned home, the telephone was ringing. My husband answered it, and I saw his expression change and heard his voice fall. Dr. K was on the line. He said he knew we would want to hear the results right away. There were sarcoma cells in the mass on his liver. Our worst fears were realized.

How could this be? Barry felt so good! He looked the picture of health, and the PET scan had shown no cancer at all. We thought we had beaten this cancer. How many times could this happen? How many times would our emotions see-saw between hope and despair? Dr. K was suggesting the experimental chemo treatment he was developing, which was now about to be used in Phase 3 of a trial study at Sloan-Kettering. He also wanted us to schedule a consultation with Dr. B., the chief of surgery at Memorial Sloan-Kettering, and the top sarcoma expert. We knew that our own Dr. Lewis was close to Dr. B., and had consulted with him throughout Barry's treatment, so our case would not be completely new to him. We would try to meet with Dr. B. as soon as possible. Then we would decide what course to take.

We knew that it would be difficult to get an appointment with Dr. B. After all, he was the leading specialist in sarcoma, the doctor we had tried to see when Barry's tumor had first appeared. Before calling Dr. B.'s office, we decided to call our own Dr. Lewis He was, after all, still our advisor. Dr. Lewis was out of town. We didn't ordinarily call him when he was out of town, but this was a near-emergency, and after some hesitancy, Barry dialed his cell phone number. Dr. Lewis answered. He was in the middle of a meeting in Chicago, but he took the time to listen to our news. He agreed that it would be a good idea to call Dr. B. in to consult. It was time for us to meet him in person. Barry ended the conversation by asking Dr. Lewis if he could help us get a timely appointment with Dr. B. "Of course," he said. What a friend!

We met with Dr. B. and, to our surprise, our appointment with him was easy. We had not expected this renowned doctor to be so congenial and compassionate. He smiled at us as he walked into the examining room, exclaiming, "At last, you're mine!" When Dr. Lewis left Sloan, he had transferred many of his patients to Dr. B. and to Dr. B's. younger associates, but he had kept Barry and a few others for himself. Now, finally, we were also Dr. B.'s.

Dr. B. reassured us that there were several avenues of treatment open, including some surgical procedures. He smiled again, saying that Barry wouldn't get any sympathy from him; he looked too good for that. His humor eased our tension. Dr. B. told us he would carefully review my husband's record, including all the scans, then talk to Dr. K., and get back to us. We left with renewed hope. Now we understood why Dr. B. and our Dr. Lewis were close colleagues and friends; they were two of a kind.

CHAPTER TWENTY-FIVE

A NEW PLAN OF ACTION
(Feb – March '01)

D r. B. kept his word and called us back in a few days. He agreed with Dr. K. that the experimental chemo would be the best first step. If that "took care of it," as he put it, we wouldn't need to do anything else. We held onto Dr. B's words; they told us it was possible for this chemo to take care of the tumor. It was possible......

We continued to consult with Dr. Lewis, who recounted histories of his patients who had survived several surgeries, or several chemo regimens. He called this tumor of Barry's "well-behaved." He always had a story to make us feel that there was hope for us. There was always another patient who had made it through a worse situation, and was doing well. He had a big bag of tricks handy, and was ready to pull out whatever we needed.

We spoke with Dr. K. on the phone as well, and made preparations for the experimental chemo. Since we would be part of a Memorial Sloan-Kettering study, the chemo would have to be administered at that hospital in New York City. We would miss the comfort of our local hospital and the medical staff we knew so well. We would be an hour and a half from home by car, or more by train, so that if Barry felt sick after his treatments, we would face a difficult trip home. We could not know how he would feel after this new chemo, as the regimen was still being developed. But this still seemed our best choice. Before actually starting the chemotherapy, Barry would have to have a "port" installed, and register to be part of the study. The Sloan-Kettering staff helped us arrange for these things, since we were in the dark about all of these new procedures. In contrast to our work with other medical offices, Dr. K.'s staff never offered information, expressed confidence, or gave us the feeling that things would be okay.

One of the difficult things Barry had to face now, as he had before, was the prospect of becoming a patient again after months of feeling so well. Being a patient involves the loss of control, a sense of helplessness, fear of the unknown, and often, the anticipation of pain. We take so much for granted when we are well; it is such a blessing. Luckily for most people, they live life "unafflicted" most of the time. Now Barry was feeling and looking great, but we were voluntarily taking a step that would force him back into the role of patient. Soon, we knew, he might become very sick, in our effort to save his life. This was hard to do.

The mediport to be installed in his chest would be the device through which the chemo could be infused, instead of administering it intravenously in his arm, as we had done so far. When people have a lot of toxic chemotherapy treatments, or multiple courses of chemo, a port is often installed, and it prevents damage to the patient's veins.

The insertion of the mediport was scheduled to be done at Mt. Sinai Hospital, where we could arrange an appointment sooner than at Sloan-Kettering. We arrived early, and when they ushered us into the "interventional radiology" area, we found ourselves sitting on two chairs in a hallway. Nearby was an elderly man lying on a stretcher. A young woman in dungarees, apparently a radiology resident, came out of a room to take a history from the man on the stretcher; not a private interview, but right there in the hall. Soon she did the same with us. As Barry recounted his history, she looked at him in amazement. I am sure no resident was ever given such a complete medical account. Then Barry was taken into the procedure room, and I was left to wait the hour or so in the hallway. Eventually, one of the radiologists showed me another area where families could wait, an alcove out of the narrow and crowded hall. Once the mediport was installed, we were on our way home. Barry was alert after the procedure, as he had not been sedated. He had no trouble walking back to the car, and as I drove us home, his local anesthetic was still in effect, and he was comfortable.

On our way home, we decided to stop at our office to see if the staff needed us for anything. Barry was feeling fine, not sore yet from the procedure. As it turned out, there was a young man with an emergency, who needed to be seen. We had him come right over, and Barry examined him before we continued on our way home. As the teenage patient left the office, his mother turned to us and said, "Well, enjoy the rest of your day off." When she had called the office earlier, our secretary had told her that the doctor was "out for the day," but would call her later. It appeared to her that Barry had the day off, when he had really spent it as a patient in another hospital.

As we approached home, the local anesthetic was beginning to wear off. I could see Barry wincing and holding his chest where the port had been inserted. We were home just in the nick of time. We realized then that nobody had told us how to take care of the two wounds in Barry's neck and chest, how and when to change the dressings, and what to do or to avoid. Being a physician, my husband knew what to do, but what on earth would an ordinary patient do in this situation?

The following week we had a CAT scan scheduled, along with an appointment with Dr. K. to register us for the chemo study. It would be a busy week.

CHAPTER TWENTY-SIX

A WEEK TO FORGET
(March '01)

Barry rested a lot on the weekend after his mediport was put in; he certainly wasn't up to doing any physical work. He wasn't in pain, but he wasn't completely comfortable, either. It took some adjusting to have holes in your chest and neck, and to know that a tube was inside connecting them under your skin. Beneath the incision in Barry's chest, the mediport protruded as a round bump under the skin. At this site needles would be inserted to deliver the chemo drugs. We hoped there would come a time when the port could be removed.

The Sunday after the port procedure, the weather forecasters predicted that the winter storm of the decade was about to hit the East Coast. Every weatherman was positive that this storm would drop enormous amounts of snow on the New York metropolitan area, taking out power lines in many communities. Schools and businesses were canceling Monday operations in advance.

On Sunday afternoon, I called the Monday patients for our office to cancel their appointments. Many of our patients were older, and wouldn't want to drive in bad weather anyway, and I didn't want to have to call people very early on Monday morning. Then Barry and I prepared for the storm to hit. By Sunday night the forecasters were saying that the storm might be slow in arriving, but that once it started, it would snow all day and night Monday and into Tuesday, leading people to believe that Tuesday morning might be worse than Monday. When Monday morning rolled around and the snow was still light, I realized that if it hit on Tuesday, we might not get to our scheduled CAT scan. I called our local hospital to see if we could have it done on Monday instead. It turned out to be a great idea: the hospital had cancelled all the Monday scans, so the schedule was wide open. We had already picked up the barium Barry needed for the scan, so we were all set. Barry drank the barium, and we jumped in the car, put it in four wheel drive, and made our way through the snow to the hospital, where we got the CAT scan performed in record time.

We had the CAT scan report faxed to Dr. K., Dr. B., and our own Dr. Lewis. This time, Barry did not request a copy for himself. He couldn't bear any more bad news.

The snow came down and came down, all day Monday, and into Tuesday. Schools were closed both days, but the local highway departments managed to keep the roads plowed. Tuesday morning, as we made our way to the train station for our appointment with Dr. K. at Memorial Sloan-Kettering, the roads were icy. Barry drove, and it took all his skill to maneuver the car as we skidded dangerously near telephone poles and trucks.

We were meeting with Dr. K. to register for Phase 3 of the experimental study. There were blood tests to be done, papers to sign, disclaimers to read, and many instructions for the weeks ahead. The chemotherapy treatments would start the following week. All of our doctors had agreed that this was Barry's best chance to stop the tumor on his liver. Dr. K. was pleased that all was in order, and even smiled at us as we left. We were to see him exactly one week later, early in the morning, and we were prepared to spend most of the day at Sloan, getting the first dose of the new miracle chemo drug.

As we waited for the elevator on our way out of the hospital, one of Dr. K.'s young assistants came over to us and asked us to wait a minute before we left; Dr. K. wanted to see us again. Puzzled, we walked back into the exam room to wait. This time when the doctor walked in, he wasn't smiling. He spoke bluntly, "You don't qualify for the study. Your blood test shows a bilirubin level that is too high to participate." Rejected. Period. No other options; no suggestions. We were stunned. We asked whether we could repeat the blood test. Dr. K. said we should do it right then and there, and he would call us later that evening with the results.

We went home to wait for a phone call. At 6:00 PM Dr. K. called. He was still at work. The second test showed a bilirubin level of 1.1. This was lower than the first test but still one-tenth of one percent too high for the study. *One-tenth of one percent!* Barry, desperately trying to save his life, asked if the test could be performed once more, the following day at our local hospital. Dr. K. agreed. So, early the next morning, Barry stopped at the hospital on his way to the office, and repeated the test. The level of bilirubin read 0.8! We faxed the results to Dr. K.'s office, confident that Barry qualified for the study now.

We tried to have a relaxing weekend, but it was hard with an unknown chemotherapy regimen looming. We didn't know what to expect in terms of side-effects or how sick Barry would feel. He had become subdued; his step was slower. He seemed to be turning inwards. I decided we needed a treat: I got us ice-cream.

Dr. Lewis called us on Sunday afternoon about another matter; but he was so encouraging about Barry's prognosis that he cheered us both up. He said that he thought this treatment would work, and that there were other options available to us if we needed them. How could you feel depressed or negative when you had a man like this behind you? When I said that I didn't know how to thank him, he replied, in his modest way, "You already have."

Barry and I were both surprised on Monday afternoon when Dr. K.'s assistant called us at home. She was checking on what chemo my husband had already been given. This information was in his Sloan-Kettering record; was she double-checking? We told her about the two prior courses of chemo, but we thought to ourselves, *Why couldn't they read the record?* We asked if things were in order for the following day. "Yes," she said.

Early that evening, I answered the phone. Dr. K. was calling. His voice was flat. "I won't be able to give your husband the chemo tomorrow; his application has been rejected for the study." I couldn't believe my ears! How could this be happening? I quickly gave the telephone to Barry. He was as stunned as I was. I heard him arguing with Dr. K.; arguing for his life. He needed this drug. Apparently, this phase of the chemo study was open only to people who had had at least three prior courses of chemo drugs; my husband had had only two. Again, he didn't fit the criteria for the study. It was cut and dry. There was no leeway. What could we do? We saw the best possible treatment being snatched away from us. We were devastated.

I listened as Barry asked what we should do. I could see he was distraught. Dr. K. was saying there were other drugs Barry could try, but they were not very effective. "And they have severe side effects," he added. Finally, Dr. K. said that he could apply for what was called "compassionate use" of the experimental drug. Two committees had to approve its use; one was in Spain. Barry said he would consult with Dr. B. and Dr. Lewis and decide what to do. Did we have any choices left? Dr. K. made everything sound hopeless. How ironic that we needed a man who seemed so devoid of feeling to seek "compassionate use" for us....

Barry hung up the phone and immediately called Dr. B.'s office. Dr. B. said he would talk to Dr. K. He said we could reach him at his office the following afternoon, as he would be in surgery all morning. To our surprise, he said it was usually not difficult to get approval for compassionate use. *Why couldn't Dr. K. have told us that?*

Next Barry called Dr. Lewis's office. Dr. Lewis was en route from Boston to New York, but his secretary said she could get a message to him. Then we sat down together and tried to calm ourselves. We had to be strong now. Sure enough, Dr. Lewis called as soon as he landed in New York. Barry told him his situation, and Dr. Lewis agreed that the experimental drug was the best choice for us now, and we should wait for Dr. K. to get compassionate use approval. He, too, said it was usually not a problem to obtain. That gave us some relief.

There had been several times during this illness when panic had set in, and when both Barry and I felt hopeless, and full of fear. It was like being on heightened alert, as in any emergency. By now we knew that this state didn't last forever; it was self-limiting. The first time it had happened, two and a half years earlier, Barry had been talking to a friend in the locker room of our swimming club, a man who practiced psychiatry. This man had assured Barry that the mind couldn't sustain panic indefinitely, and that as a person relaxes, he adjusts to the new condition. That information was comforting at the time, and it stuck with us. It helped to know that even though we were in a state of alarm, our minds would take care of it and eventually we would relax.

CHAPTER TWENTY-SEVEN

WAITING
(Mar '01)

It had been almost three years since the appearance of the sarcoma. We had tried all the known treatments, and now all we could do was to wait for permission to get the experimental drug. Wait with our hearts in our mouths. And try to remain as calm and as healthy as possible.

We had some extra time that first week, since we had cleared all appointments from the office schedule for the chemotherapy treatments we thought we would be getting at Sloan. We used our free time to drive to the beach sanctuary, and even though it was early March and chilly, it was wonderful. We took walks, and gave ourselves time for naps. I usually hated to take naps, but when faced with extreme stress, I found that I needed them. So I was learning to listen to my body, and not to fight it. It really helped somehow. I continued with my swimming. Barry and I were both swimmers, but he had to wait until the incisions for his port were healed before he returned to the pool with me. I also went to my karate class, which helped mentally as well as physically. I had started practicing karate years earlier, when one of my daughters suggested we learn it together. When she dropped it, I had continued, intrigued by the mental and spiritual side of the sport, as well as the physical. My Sensei was a true master and an inspiring teacher. Under his instruction I found myself doing moves that I would never have believed possible. That itself was a confidence builder and cheered me on with my other battle.

And so the week passed. We created diversions to keep our minds from continuously focusing on the waiting, and on the terrible fear that perhaps the approval would not be granted after all. On the weekend, it was harder to keep ourselves distracted. We considered going away for the weekend, but we both were too preoccupied. I could tell that Barry was gradually succumbing to the stress. I rarely saw him smile any more.

On Sunday, I suggested that we go to New York City, visit a museum, and perhaps see our daughter, Ellen. That seemed to perk him up. It turned out to be a great day.

We browsed in the Metropolitan Museum bookstore, waiting for Ellen to meet us. I was reaching for a book on Dali, when a voice behind me warned, "Ah, don't touch that!" When I turned around, there was my daughter, grinning! I was so happy to see her and to see that she still had her sense of humor. By the time we found Barry in another aisle of the bookstore, we were laughing too hard to pull the same trick on him. The three of us strolled through the museum for hours, until we were exhausted. There were many new exhibits, and we especially enjoyed returning to the primitive artifacts, the 20th century painting, the medieval coats of armor, the early American furniture, and the Egyptian mummies. We sat for a long time by the Temple of Dendur, enjoying some people-watching, which was almost as interesting as the exhibits. After we rested, we drove Ellen downtown to a meeting she had scheduled, and on the way home took a detour through the east side neighborhood where Barry had gone to medical school. That busy and wonderful day took his mind off the worries at hand.

We entered the second week of waiting. We could do nothing now except try to be patient and have faith in our doctors. Barry had office hours in the mornings, and we took time for walks in the afternoons. I went to karate class, and felt comfort and support from the other students as well as from my kind teacher. I recall telling him how we had been notified of the chemo cancellation the night before it was supposed to start. He shook his head. "Ahhhhh, no respect," he said. How true.

In a few days, Barry felt ready to try swimming again. He was self-conscious about the bump in his chest created by the port under the skin. I was more concerned that his vigorous swimming stroke might dislodge the port from its connection. But all went well, and he enjoyed both the return to the exercise and the camaraderie of the early morning swimmers. We were a friendly group of people who all enjoyed the ridiculous routine of getting up at the crack of dawn, driving through the semi-darkness, and jumping into a cold swimming pool before we had even wiped the sleep out of our eyes. We were old, young, super-fast swimmers and slow-paddlers, retirees and those rushing off to work; fat, thin; old, bent over with arthritis and young and sleek. We all appreciated the company of the other early risers, and shared each others' stories of life's ups and downs. I must say that for me the best part of swimming was climbing out of the pool when I was done; that felt so good. The hardest part was jumping into the cold water!

After swimming, we went to work at our office, keeping one ear open for a call from Dr. K. It did not come. I planned to call Dr. K. that afternoon, if we didn't hear from him by then. We saw our morning patients, then left the office to do errands and go home. No sooner had we left the office, than Barry's beeper went off. It was our secretary. Dr. K. had called, and she knew how much we were anticipating his call. We returned the call immediately. Dr. K. said that he had obtained approval to use the drug on Barry, and would start treatment the following Tuesday. We were elated. Only then did I realize how scared I had been that Dr. K. might fail to get the okay for the chemo. If approval were denied, we would have had absolutely no recourse. This drug was being developed privately, and could be withheld on the whim of the company doing the research. They were accountable to nobody in this decision, and did not have to make the drug available outside the study. Now we could get this precious medicine, and treatment would begin soon!

Suddenly there was so much to do. We were grabbing a quick bite of lunch before heading back to the office, when Barry turned to me with alarm. He said that I was as white as a sheet. I could feel my heart racing. I had been trying to stay calm, but I couldn't adjust to the huge emotional swings from hopelessness to fear, to relief, and, dare I say it, hope again? But I had tried to appear relaxed so I wouldn't get Barry even more upset. We were so happy to be able to get the drug, yet so scared of what lay ahead. We dreaded being back in the hospital setting, at the mercy of doctors and nurses we didn't know. *It's an amazing thing: you dread getting the poisonous chemo, but the moment it is being withheld from you, you beg for it.....*

Back at the office, I had to cancel Barry's appointments for the following week and reschedule them for a future date. *How many times could we do this to our patients?* I also had a list of people to call and notify; I did what I could, and left instructions at the office for our secretary to do the rest. Then we went home.

We spent the rest of the week preparing for the chemo. Barry said again he felt that time was running out. So many times he had been brought to the brink and then stepped back. Nobody knew just what this chemo could do; in its previous trials, it had seemed effective. But what did that mean? Did it get rid of the tumor, or just slow its growth? Did you take it for several months, or, as we feared, forever? And what had happened in the past when patients had stopped the treatment? We were afraid to ask Dr. K. No sense in making ourselves pessimistic. We needed all the hope we could muster right now. So we pushed fear to the back of our minds, and went about the business of doing what had to be done, and then trying to have fun. I guess that sounds ridiculous.

CHAPTER TWENTY-EIGHT

ANOTHER DELAY
(March '01)

On Saturday of that weekend, we decided to take a drive over to our favorite beach along the Connecticut shore. It was chilly, but we enjoyed that place so much that we decided to go anyway. Soon after we got there, the sun disappeared behind clouds, but the spot was peaceful, and there were flocks of birds along the beach and in the woods to cheer us. This was a nature sanctuary, and we often saw beautiful birds such as loons, egrets and swans. We had brought the video camera to tape the scenery for our daughter in Alaska. We often did that sort of thing for her, and she and her husband taped the scenery around Fairbanks to send to us, to show us parts of their world.

We strolled along the paths and trails, videotaping the clouds, the birds, Long Island Sound, the windblown trees. After a while, a few raindrops began to fall, and we started to increase our pace, heading back toward the car. The wind picked up, and the rain came faster and faster. By the time we reached the protection of our Jeep, we were wet and freezing. The cold rain had been coming down horizontally. It was strange: the left side of my face was cold and wet, but the right side was dry and warm. There were many other wet souls, caught out in the elements, seeking shelter under the trees, or running back to their cars. I thought this was great fun; it was the kind of venture I loved. Barry was less enthusiastic; he didn't relish a walk in the rain; he never had.

Once home and inside the house, we saw our answering machine blinking; what could this be? We heard Dr. K.'s voice on the message, warning us of another delay in the start of the chemo. This was truly unbelievable! Dr. K. was apologizing; he could not give us the chemo this week, because the drug had not been shipped from the company on time. Another postponement. Would all this delay lessen the chances that the drug would work by the time Barry finally got it? Nobody knew.

We told ourselves that our situation was not that bad. This was just a delay of a week or so, not a rejection or denial of the experimental drug. What could we do, anyway? We were at the mercy of some unknown foreign company manufacturing and shipping the drug.

We spent the rest of the weekend trying to adapt to one more change. Barry did hours of yard work in the crisp March air. He had never lived in a house until we bought our first one, many years earlier. He loved to make minor repairs and had learned about electrical and plumbing systems. But it was the outdoor work that provided the greatest pleasure for him, and now it was a release for his stress. He pruned bushes and cut small tree limbs, dragging them into the woods. The weather was chilly but the sun was shining. Barry enjoyed getting the land ready for spring, and the physical exercise strengthened and invigorated him. Every time he came inside, his cheeks were flushed and he was breathless. He was really getting a work-out, and we both were appreciative that he could still do this. He wanted to do everything he possibly could to keep up the property in case we should need to sell it. That was another unspoken fear.

Later, when we drove into town to pick up Chinese food for dinner, we enjoyed the late winter landscape. The trees were bare, but we could see the buds getting ready to pop open. The sun was higher in the sky; birds were coming back; somehow you just knew that before long things would be breaking out in bloom. A few perennials were beginning to poke up through the cold earth. We had been driving for about ten minutes when I realized that I had left the kettle on the stove! *Had I really done that?* I thought so, or had I returned to the kitchen and turned it off, as I had intended to do? I couldn't remember at all! This was a sign of my growing distraction. I had been trying to stay calm, but, day after day, I was beginning to do more and more things that I didn't mean to do, or forgetting what I had done. As you can imagine, I was distraught as we drove through town, picked up the food, and returned to the house. The kitchen was intact: no fire, no smoke, just a dry, scorched kettle, and a lousy smell. Again, I determined to pay careful attention to what I was doing, and not to let the stress of our situation create any additional problems!

Actually, there was a different concern in the back of my mind. I had just had a check-up with my gynecologist, and he had seen something suspicious. He had taken a biopsy and was to call me with the results as soon as he had them. He was a superb and careful doctor and a compassionate man, and I had the utmost confidence in him. And he was going through a situation similar to mine: his wife had cancer, and it had been discovered at roughly the same time as my husband's. Often, after my exams, we would exchange stories, half-afraid to ask how the other's spouse was doing.

CHAPTER TWENTY-NINE

HEALTH INSURANCE

Everyone assumes that doctors and their families have great health insurance. Surprisingly, this is not always true. Our family had always had health insurance through Barry's professional association, and it had been with the same insurance company for many years. It was expensive, but it had served us well, both before his illness and then, more importantly, during his cancer treatment.

Out of the blue, during the previous fall, we had received a letter from the insurance company, telling us that their rates were going up. We weren't pleased, but these days that was to be expected. I scanned the sheet with the details, looking for the category with our age and location. I couldn't believe my eyes: the rate listed was almost ten times the previous rate! There had to be an error here; perhaps this was the annual rate, not the monthly rate. We called the company, and learned that the rates were correct as listed. We couldn't believe it.

Barry called his professional academy next; they were unaware of the situation. How could they not know that their own members' health insurance was becoming unaffordable? We paid dues to this group for precisely this purpose. The academy told us that the insurance company was trying to get out of their contract with the association, and within a year or so the rates would be prohibitive. We knew we would have to start looking for new health insurance. Just another headache, along with all the others we had.

We began investigating insurance, consulting with insurance companies directly, and with agents as well. Since we didn't need new coverage immediately, we could carefully consider whatever policies were available to individuals. With our old coverage, we hadn't needed referrals for every test and exam we had. It would be hard to find another policy like that; in the future, we would probably have to get approval for each scan, test, consultation and treatment we needed. I dreaded that prospect. All we could do was hope that we could find a liberal policy. This would take time and energy; and we would just have to deal with it - as soon as we got the problem with the chemo treatments underway. There were only so many situations I could handle at one time. I filed this away for future consideration.

During this period, a multitude of issues swirled through my mind at once: thoughts about Barry's treatment, medical insurance, our children, my future, Barry's future, his medical practice. Wherever I turned, I hit a brick wall. It was hard to understand how my life had changed so much in what seemed like such a short time. What I had considered normal was long gone; all my expectations had changed.

I had always looked forward to a long and healthy life with my husband. When we met, I was eighteen and Barry was twenty. We were full of hope and optimism; who isn't at that age? We had been ready to work hard to build a good life. And we had. We had two wonderful children, a warm extended family, a comfortable home, good friends, and Barry's thriving practice. And it had not been all work; we had enjoyed many trips to special places that we found spiritual and inspiring. We loved the same sorts of vacations, and we learned to adjust.

As young adults, when we had looked ahead into the future, and thought about the turn of the century, actually, the "millennium," it seemed light years away. Now it had come and gone. We were still here, still together, but engaged in the battle of our lives.

CHAPTER THIRTY

Waiting for Chemo

It was the last week in March. We were working for just one more week, before the day the experimental chemo would start. Our tentative date was the following Tuesday, with a return appointment on Wednesday to have the portable chemo pump "disconnected." Whatever that meant. We had never seen one of these pumps, and could only imagine what it would be like. Bulky? Noisy? My mind conjured up pictures of big, complicated machines.

On the way home from work, we stopped at our local hospital, where Barry picked up the papers from his box in the doctors' mailroom. One of these was the report of the CAT scan that had been done three weeks earlier. This was the scan for the chemo study, the one we had chosen not to see. Now, Barry hurried to the car with the report in his hand and a worried look on his face. The report noted that there were several new lesions on his liver. In addition, the one that they had been watching all these months had grown. Barry felt that he was doomed. This news was dire. Barry was terrified. We drove home in silence.

That afternoon we called Dr. Lewis. We couldn't remember whether we had sent him the CAT scan report or not. Dr. Lewis said that the new lesions were small, and could be dealt with. He also told us that there were other options, before it would be necessary to consider surgery. At least he wasn't telling Barry to get his affairs in order and to prepare for the end. We trusted this man to never give us false hope. His words quieted our immediate fears.

We hung up the phone and it rang again. It was my own doctor, calling with the results of my biopsy from the previous week. He was pleased to report that the tests were negative. His news hardly registered with me; I was so upset about Barry's situation that I couldn't grasp the significance this report. Only later did the relief hit me. I realized how worried I had been. *How*

could we cope if I suddenly needed treatment or surgery? I was
supposed to be the care-giver. But life doesn't give you problems
neatly, lining them up so you can deal with them one at a time.

With the chemo scheduled for some time in the coming week,
and no information from Dr. K.'s office, Barry and I began to fear
his case was falling through the cracks. We were sinking into a rut,
unable to stay hopeful. For the first time in this entire experience,
we started snapping at each other. I felt that I could handle whatever
came our way, but I could not handle it if we began taking out our
frustrations on each other. I could see that Barry was despondent,
feeling as if there was no hope left. I knew that Dr. Lewis wouldn't
string us along, if there truly were no hope, but Barry was so scared
that my words made no impact. I was getting more and more upset. I
said I couldn't fight this disease by myself, that he could not give up.
But it wasn't my life, was it? I wasn't the one with the lesions growing
inside of me. We went to bed that night, but didn't sleep much, and I
woke up with a sore throat. It was a dark morning indeed.

That weekend, the weather matched our mood; it was gray,
drizzly and cold. I felt I had a virus, and worried that I would give
it to Barry, jeopardizing his treatment. I spent a lot of time sleeping;
he spent that time worrying.

On Sunday afternoon I asked Barry to go out to pick up
dinner, since I wasn't up to cooking, and I was afraid I would
give him my virus if I prepared the food. As soon as he left, Dr.
Lewis called. He let us know that he had heard from a chemo
nurse at Sloan that Dr. K.'s team was "making every effort" to
get the drug for us this week. He couldn't promise, of course,
and he knew what hardship we had already been through with
broken promises, but he thought chances were good. When we
hung up, I burst into tears. This man was so compassionate, I
couldn't thank him enough. He gave us hope when we had none,
caring when nobody else had a kind word to say. With hope, you
can withstand anything, but without hope, you just don't have
the strength. When Barry got home, I was hopeful, peaceful, and
smiling, although my eyes were red. We just couldn't get over
how lucky we were to have such a great person behind us.

CHAPTER THIRTY-ONE

WOULD WE GET THE CHEMO?
(April '01)

It was April: springtime, Daylight Savings Time, opening day at Yankee Stadium, with longer days, and warmer temperatures, although this year they were well below normal. We could hear birds singing in the early mornings, and the Canada geese were flying north. The deer were back, nipping the new buds from our bushes. Passover was almost upon us, and again I didn't feel up to making a Seder. If we were able to get the first dose of the new chemo this week, there would be no way to have a family get-together at all. It had been exactly two years since Barry had begun his first course of chemotherapy. And now we were waiting to hear whether we would be able to have more of the life-saving poison delivered for us. Even if our prayers were answered, and the drug did arrive, nobody knew whether it would be effective. But that hurdle was sometime in the future.

All Monday morning, while seeing patients in our office, we kept an ear open for the promised call from Dr. K.'s office. It did not come. Finally, at the end of the morning, the phone rang and we heard that the drug was being shipped that very day, and would arrive on Tuesday. We could start on Wednesday. Dr. K. actually thanked us for our patience. We were elated: we had a definite date! We would be able to get the chemo! The dreaded chemo......the desperately needed chemo.....

One of our patients that morning was the wife of a man with cancer, whom we had known for years. They were currently preparing for his third stem cell transplant. They had these done at Mayo Clinic in Minneapolis, where they went and stayed for a month each time. This man had been treated for years for a disease that had been expected to kill him long ago. Still he was living, working, enjoying his grandchildren. When he came to our office, we would compare notes; sometimes he was bald, sometimes Barry was; sometimes he was between treatments, sometimes we were. In the midst of all this, his wife developed breast cancer, and I saw her at the supermarket on the last day of her chemo. She had lost her hair, but was happy to report that she was finished with her treatment. I wondered how I would deal with something like that. It took all of my strength to deal with my husband's disease. *How on earth did people deal with another burden on top of that?*

Meanwhile, I was trying desperately to keep Barry from catching my cold. What a terrible time for me to get a virus. We now had one full day to prepare ourselves for the experimental chemo. We tried not to worry that something else would go wrong with the arrangements.

I spent the day at home. I rested, did paperwork, and tried to relax and pamper myself and my cold. I knew I needed to be ready to be the driver, the caregiver, the protector. Barry, meanwhile, was living on nervous energy. He was dreading becoming a patient again. He went to the office, dealt with office business, spoke to patients who called, did some errands, and later, at home, did some physical yard work. He was driven by the sense that his time was running out. That was not Dr. Lewis's message to us, but I understood how Barry could feel this way. We ate dinner quietly, both of us dreading a call from Dr. K., announcing one more delay. I watched the minutes tick by, knowing that as they did, it became less likely that our appointment would be cancelled. Finally, we went to bed, but I was still praying the phone would not ring.

When we woke up the next morning, and the cancellation hadn't happened, we jumped out of bed and headed for Memorial Sloan-Kettering, with hope in our hearts despite the odds.

CHAPTER THIRTY-TWO

A NEW REGIMEN

The procedure for the experimental chemo was entirely new to us. We were grateful to be getting the new drug, but we were also unnerved by the complicated process it entailed. The medication was to be delivered over a 24-hour period. This would involve going home with a portable pump and a cassette of the drug, and returning to Sloan-Kettering the following day to have the pump disconnected when delivery of the dose was complete.

We began the treatment with an early morning visit to Dr. K., in the uptown Sloan facility. Then we boarded the MSKCC mini-van that shuttled patients and staff from the hospital to the Sloan-Kettering outpatient facility on 53rd Street. We checked in at the chemo department at 10:30 AM, thinking we were ready for whatever this experience would bring. But we were not prepared for the four-hour delay that followed.

We waited and waited, returning to the check-in desk from time to time to ask if everything was all right, and the reason for the delay. Nobody knew what was causing the delay, but the pharmacy was backed up and had not sent the drug up to the chemo department. The facility was swamped with patients. When the drug finally arrived, we were ushered into a chemo room, and the nurses started the procedure. They cleaned the port in Barry's chest three times and gave him the pre-chemo medications. But now there was another delay. Dr. K.'s approval was needed to deliver the drugs through Barry's port, rather than through a vein. The doctor's orders were not specific enough.

Finally, at 2:30 PM, one of the nurses walked into our exam room, holding a cassette with Barry's medicine. I was struck by the number of times the nurses checked and double-checked the medication, the dose, and the orders from the doctor. No mistakes could be tolerated. We watched a video about using the portable pump, and what to do if it failed, if its battery failed, or if a line got kinked. Now we were ready to head home - numb and drained.

As we rode in the Sloan van back to our car at the uptown MSKCC building, Barry's beeper went off. Our secretary was calling to ask him about a patient who needed advice. It was surreal to be sitting in a van hooked up to a chemo pump, one of many cancer patients stuck in New York City traffic, talking to our secretary about a patient's pinkeye. Soon our van stopped cold behind an oil truck that was making a delivery to an apartment building. We sat on that side-street until the truck had filled the entire oil tank for this large building. Talk about ridiculous!

At last, we were back in our own car, headed home, nervous about the new pump, and listening for warning beeps it might emit. I drove slowly, hoping Barry would not get carsick, since one of the side-effects of the medicine was nausea. But as we made our way out of the city into the suburbs with more trees and grass, we began to relax a little. It was good to get back to the comfort of our own home. We went to bed early, listening all night for beeps warning of trouble with the pump.

Our appointment the following day was at 2:30 P.M., exactly twenty-four hours after the treatment had been started. This time there was no waiting. Within a short time, the pump was disconnected and Barry was given his post-chemo drugs and dismissed. We were out in the street, released into the real world. After the intensive period of treatment, we felt cut loose, set adrift. We tried to remember what "normal" was again.

Every time you complete a chemo dose, there is elation that you have done something positive, that there is medicine inside you that is working to destroy the cancer. However slight, there is hope.

Driving home, we felt great. We trusted the medicine to do its job. We were free for a few weeks and spring was in the air. As we drove up the East River Drive, I listened to the traffic report on the radio. It was nearing rush hour and the announcer said that the ballgame at Yankee Stadium was in its ninth inning. We would have to hurry to miss the traffic exiting from the stadium. As we approached the Triborough Bridge, the game ended, and the Yankees had won. The stands would be emptying out; hundreds or thousands of fans would be streaming out of the parking lots and onto the highway. There was nothing we could do but keep on driving. When we reached Yankee Stadium, we were in the midst of the traffic, but who cared?

CHAPTER THIRTY-THREE

AFTER-EFFECTS

Barry now had to deal with the side effects of the chemo, and we both had to rest and recuperate. Make no mistake about it: the caregiver needs to recuperate almost as much as the patient. Almost. There were required post-chemo blood tests to get at our local hospital. In two days it would be Passover and it was also my birthday. We had no plan for a Seder or celebration this year. We were exhausted, and relieved to have this first treatment over with, to have the experimental medicine at last. Now at least we knew what was involved, and what to expect next time.

Ellen was planning to come up from New York City over the weekend, but we wouldn't be seeing any other family. I felt protective of my mother - I didn't want her to see Barry, or me, for that matter, in such an exhausted condition. We ended up having a very nice weekend. We shared my birthday ice-cream cake with Ellen in a modest celebration. Barry was still on a tapered-down dose of steroid, which made him energetic, and the full side-effects of the chemo were not yet in evidence. We were grateful that he didn't seem to be getting nauseous from the treatment.

As the weekend wore on, Barry became more and more exhausted from the drug. I followed his symptoms and noted them in our chemo log. Two years earlier, our chemo nurse had advised us to keep a notebook with details of how each drug affected him and what side effects occurred, such as nausea, tiredness, or weakness. Every time Barry had a new chemo drug, I diligently recorded these data. We found it helpful to refer to this log, as we couldn't keep track of all these details without a written record.

As I eased back into daily activities, I watched for signs that Barry's energy was returning. *How strange it is to feel far removed from all normal activities while you are receiving treatment, and to dip your toes tentatively back into life again between treatments.*

Barry described the feeling as having a curtain separating him from the rest of the world.

It was a full week after the end of the chemo dose before I could see an improvement in Barry's condition. He was able to do a little outdoor work, which amazed me. As his physical stamina improved, so did his mental state. He wanted to be as active as he could, to feel normal. Nobody likes to feel like a helpless, dependent patient. By the time we spoke to Dr. Lewis, we could both report that we were doing well. Dr. Lewis repeated his encouragement, underscoring how promising the early reports of the new drug had been.

We arrived at Sloan-Kettering the following Tuesday for the chemo treatment, more prepared to deal with whatever side-effects came our way. But that morning's blood tests showed that Barry's blood counts were too low to receive the medication. Dr. K. gave us the bad news, and scheduled us for another attempt the following week.

We returned home disappointed but determined to rescue the rest of the week if we could. First, we had to "come down" from the heightened state we were in, anticipating the treatment. We did the best we could, rescheduling appointments in our own office. *Life has so many little tasks that are hard to fit into a chemo schedule.* We decided to be optimistic about the blood counts returning to acceptable levels, and planned to get the chemo the next week, not thinking about the possibility that we could be turned down again.

CHAPTER THIRTY-FOUR

MORE CHEMO
(May '01)

The following week, Barry was able to receive the second dose of the experimental chemo. As before, we drove to Manhattan very early, and parked uptown at the Sloan-Kettering garage. But this time Barry felt well enough to walk to the outpatient facility on 53rd Street, through the early morning hustle-bustle of the city. Dr. K. seemed pleased to hear how well Barry had tolerated the treatment: no nausea, no sick feeling, just the expected fatigue. The doctor almost smiled.

As we waited to be called in for the treatment, we observed another family scene in the waiting room. A young couple had brought their elderly mother or grandma for treatment. She looked frail, and they sat and waited with her for a long time. Finally, a young receptionist approached them. There had been a mix-up, she said. Someone had neglected to inform them that their grandma could not be treated that day because her lab results had not been received. As the story unfolded, it appeared that the oncology staff had neglected to inform the family of this, and the patient had been inconvenienced, perhaps endangered. The elderly patient was despondent; her granddaughter was furious. The two young people had taken time off from work to make the trip to Sloan-Kettering. Now there was nothing to do except to go home. The receptionist offered to summon a "Patient Representative" to hear their story, but the young woman said she was far too angry to talk to anyone just then. *How many times had this scene already happened? And how many more times would it be repeated?*

Finally it was time for Barry to get his medication, and we were ushered into a chemo room. It wasn't long before we found ourselves standing outside in the sunshine again, with Barry hooked up to a chemo pump hanging over his shoulder. The Sloan-Kettering shuttle bus chauffeured us back to the uptown parking facility, and slowly we made our way home. The second dose of medicine was running through my husband's veins, and I was grateful. The following day, after a night of praying that the pump didn't malfunction, we made the return trip to the city for the disconnection. The second dose was complete. Two doses now were, hopefully, doing their job on the cancer.

The next couple of weeks were very busy for us. The after-effects of the chemo continued to be just fatigue and weakness. Barry had his usual follow-up blood tests at our local hospital. I had to have some dental work done, which turned into more than I had bargained for: a crown, a root canal procedure, and several fillings. In the midst of all this, I received a phone call from a museum that was interested in seeing my artwork. This was exciting for us both, and led to welcome distraction in the middle of all our medical and dental appointments. We visited my mother on Mother's Day, bringing her flowers and gifts, and I received presents and flowers from my grown children. For the first time in months, Barry felt good enough to attend a meeting of his department at our hospital. In addition to all of this, Ellen's theatre company was awarded a major grant, and she began intensive rehearsals for a play she was directing that was about to open. I began to think about planning a short road trip to New England, which we could slip in between chemo doses.

In the midst of all these activities, Barry and I were each trying to keep our minds off the approaching CAT scan. The results would tell us whether or not the experimental drug was affecting his tumor. We avoided mentioning the subject, each aware that the other was thinking about it. As the date for the scan approached, we became more and more nervous, but still tried to live normally. Barry told me that he felt scared about the scan, and thought that his days were numbered. This tumor was so tenacious. I tried to give him strength by repeating the positive things the doctors had told us about this chemotherapy. The early reports had been quite good. Both Dr. Lewis and Dr. B. had suggested that Barry had a number of good years left. Even Dr. K. said that this drug was most effective against the specific tumor that my husband had.

When the day of the CAT scan dawned, we drove to our local hospital quietly, as to an executioner. We didn't know when we would hear the results of this scan, or who would deliver the news. All we could do was to wait and try to calm our nerves.

CHAPTER THIRTY-FIVE

CAT SCAN RESULTS

The CAT scan was done on a Monday, and a preliminary report was faxed to our three doctors, Dr. K., Dr. Lewis, and Dr. B., that same day. We waited for news. At 9:30 that evening, Dr. Lewis called to tell us that he had been away from his office all day at meetings. He hadn't seen his faxes, but would call us as soon as he had read the report and had spoken to Dr. K. about the results. We went to bed filled with apprehension.

The week was a difficult one for us: one of waiting, keeping our phone line free, and then waiting some more. Worrying, and trying to second-guess the doctors. *Why weren't we hearing from them? Did they have to consult with each other, or hadn't they all received the reports?* By Wednesday, Barry said that if Dr. Lewis had good news, he would have called us immediately. In my heart, I had to agree with him. This delay could only mean that Dr. Lewis needed to consult with the other doctors in order to present us with any hopeful options.

Finally, on Wednesday afternoon, I went over to our hospital to get a copy of the report myself. It was supposed to have been put in Barry's mailbox at the hospital on Monday, but it still wasn't there. I went to the radiology department and was able to obtain a copy. I was so nervous reading it that I couldn't see straight. I couldn't concentrate on the medical terminology. I skimmed to the last line: there were two new lesions in the lungs, several new ones in both lobes of the liver, and the old lesion in the liver had grown. The lungs had been clean for almost two years now; how could there be new lesions in the lungs? This experimental chemo had done nothing. Nothing at all. I tried not to panic as I carried the report out to Barry, who was waiting in the hospital lobby.

How can I describe the terror of such an experience? Our hopes for remission were dashed, and our worst fears had been realized. How could the tumors be spreading when my husband looked and felt so well? It didn't make sense. And what options were left to us? We felt betrayed by this terrible disease. We returned to our car in a fog.

I know that Barry felt that he was a goner. I tried not to be so negative. I can't remember the exact sequence of events, or who called us first, but it must have been Dr. Lewis. He wanted to see us, and we arranged an appointment for two days hence. I hoped he would be able to lift our spirits somehow. When we met, he made us feel that there was still hope; he said he had seen patients with this much cancer recover with chemo. It was possible. If it had happened to others, it could happen to us. Especially since Barry's tumor had responded so well to the original chemo, two years ago. The drug they were suggesting for his next treatment was one of those he had responded to previously. More chemo. Yes, there was something we could do. We left our visit with Dr. Lewis feeling better, feeling hopeful, and feeling grateful.

We met with Dr. K., also, and were relieved to find him cordial. It seemed that the worse a patient's condition became, the more this man softened. He told us which chemo he would suggest at this point. It had the best chance of working, although it also had the most severe side effects. Both Barry and I were of the same mind: *do whatever has to be done to get rid of this cancer.* Outwardly, I was preparing for yet another round of chemo; inwardly, I was still reeling from the bad news of the CAT scan. I think I was really numb at this point.

Lifestyle questions began to loom in our minds: questions about trying to keep working versus retiring, and whether or not to remain in our house. We didn't feel able to make big decisions right then, but the issues were on our minds. Barry's actions said he was preparing to leave this world. He started dismantling his ham radio antenna, which he had done several times before, to save me the trouble. He tried to clean up loose ends in the house and yard, which I appreciated, and which also kept him busy. We both had a lot of nervous energy, yet at the same time, I felt drained.

Several events occurred just at that point which helped to take our minds off the sadness at hand. My brother and his wife were about to arrive for a short overnight visit, and their presence could help cheer us up. Our daughter's play opened at an off Broadway theatre in the city. We had been planning to see it in a few weeks, but now realized that if we didn't see it immediately, we might lose our chance. So we went into the city with a friend, and even met an aunt of my husband's who loved theatre, and made a party of the day, strolling along Spring Street and going out for dinner afterwards. The play was great, Ellen was glowing, and the day was delightful. Just what we needed.

Our last treat before returning to a difficult chemotherapy was a two day trip to Rockport, Mass., a few hours' drive north of our home. We had enjoyed Rockport years ago alone, then later with our young children, and then again by ourselves after our kids had grown up. The first time I had seen this picturesque seaport was before we were married. Barry was doing his residency in Boston, I was teaching first grade in New York City, and I had taken the train to visit him for a weekend. We had driven out to Cape Ann, where we discovered this quaint New England fishing town on the Mass. shore. Having grown up on Long Island, I loved the water. And Barry, being a city boy, found it uniquely charming. It was like stepping back in time, exploring the narrow, winding streets, with their old-fashioned shops, and then strolling barefoot on the soft, sandy beaches. Over the years, we discovered a B&B where we loved to stay, right on the main street of Rockport. At night we could lie in bed and listen to the sounds of cars passing, or in the early mornings, the milkman. This was so different from our own home on a quiet country road, where the only nighttime noises were dogs baying, and sometimes a coyote howling. We loved spending time in this little vacation spot, and it also brought up so many pleasant memories for us that it was like a rest cure.

Since this visit was spur of the moment, our usual B&B was completely booked, so we stayed at a small motel directly on the wharf. The motel windows faced west, and as dusk approached, we enjoyed a view of a gorgeous sunset, a mini-miracle from heaven. The spectacle lasted for half an hour, with colors varying from brilliant pink to orange to yellow, set off by fabulous blue-gray clouds. We returned home from this short trip restored, ready for anything.

CHAPTER THIRTY-SIX

BACK TO HEAVY CHEMO
(June '01)

June fourth, a sunny but cool Monday morning, found us driving to our local hospital, as prepared as we could be for Ifosfamide treatments, which the oncologists called "heavy-duty chemo." We were thankful to get the new treatment locally, avoiding the difficult trip to NYC. Such a concentrated dose of this medication was not often given, so nobody knew exactly what to tell us about the after-effects. We would just have to wait and see what happened. We were getting used to that.

The chemo nurses at our local hospital were wonderful; so was our local oncologist. These were people Barry had known and worked with for many years, and they were very kind to us. It really helped to make the difficult treatment manageable. But it was not just because they knew Barry that these staff members were generous; I heard them dealing with other patients, and their kindness came through with each one.

Within five hours, we were finished with the first day of the new chemo. I drove home, trying to keep the car from bouncing too much. But the day was sunny and beautiful, and the ride was fine. Barry slept for several hours; when he woke up, the nausea set in. He improved in the evening, however, and the five days of treatment passed. Before we knew it he had successfully completed the entire course of the heavy-duty Ifosfamide chemotherapy, and now we had four free weeks to look forward to.

When Barry was at home, if he was well enough to be left alone, I ventured out for my regular exercise. I appreciated resuming swimming and karate classes, especially since I hadn't expected to return to them so quickly. Whenever our medical situation became critical, all other activities had to be suspended, and I could return to them only if and when we had some time in between the medical events.

It was during the preparation for this new chemo regimen that I realized it had been three years since we had discovered the lump in Barry's leg. Three years since that fateful visit with our daughter and her husband in Seattle. Three years since we had been free of disease and worry; three years filled with surgery, radiation, procedures, CAT scans and chemo. But we had also had three years of life that Barry thought he wouldn't have. Three years to enjoy sunrises and sunsets, to enjoy being together, and to enjoy our family and friends. And to get to know, appreciate, and love the wonderful people we had met who were helping my husband to survive.

For many years, Barry had been one of those medical people helping others to survive. He had saved their vision, and even saved their lives. Now I saw and felt it all from the other side. I understood how grateful patients could be. Dealing with life and death is what had made medical training so compelling for Barry. He had always been drawn to surgery, and loved the intensity of the operating room. During his training, when he had to choose among the various surgical specialties, he had felt himself pulled in several directions. He loved the drama of orthopedics, and had almost chosen that field. Finally, working in the Public Health Service, he had discovered his love for ophthalmology. It combined the best of medicine and surgery, allowing a physician to have an office practice and ongoing personal relationships with patients, while at the same time providing the action and fulfillment of surgery. I think it was the perfect field for him. He enjoyed treating several generations of the same family, as he saw teenagers grow up, marry and then bring him children of their own. It was also gratifying for him to restore the sight of his patients, old and young, through surgery. And occasionally he would make a discovery that was life-saving, such as finding a tumor which revealed itself through subtle changes in the eye.

For the past thirty years, Barry had been one of the few ophthalmologists in our town and he had served as chief of ophthalmology at the hospital for ten of those years. He had brought the latest developments in the field to our hospital, which was becoming the preeminent facility in the area. And now he was one of the senior physicians there.

Strange.....I could close my eyes and remember his first day of medical school, not long after we had met. I was still in college, but I spent my free time visiting and studying with him and his friends at NYU. I remember his taking me up to the lab where his team was dissecting a cadaver, so excited to be seeing "the real thing." The training was arduous and they felt proud of what they were doing. Now they were scattered all across the country. So many years had gone by that most of them had lost touch with each other, yet they had been such a tight band of brothers during those four years of medical school. Now, none of them knew that Barry had been battling cancer for several years. Nobody would have believed it; he was the last person in the world that anyone would have suspected of becoming ill. Barry had always been robust and vigorous. When he and his friends had studied medicine, sarcoma had meant certain death. Now we were trying our best to believe the hope held out by our doctors that this was not always true.

Since the latest CAT scan had shown such dire evidence of Barry's disease spreading, we were losing that hope. When our daughter in Alaska heard the news, she and her husband decided to visit us. They were both teaching summer classes and taking courses themselves, but found a way to squeeze in a short visit during the Fourth of July holiday. This gave us something to look forward to while Barry was undergoing the latest chemo treatment.

Another bright spot at this time was the success Ellen was having with her new play. She was getting prominent, favorable reviews in the best papers and weeklies. People were finally beginning to notice her and her theatre company. All her hard work and determination were beginning to pay off. Barry remarked to me that he was glad he had lived long enough to see this, and I answered that he would live to see much more. Even as the available options were running out, we were trying to be optimistic. Somehow, we succeeded most of the time.

CHAPTER THIRTY-SEVEN

AFTERMATH OF HEAVY CHEMO

We had no idea what to expect during the days following the Ifosfamide treatments. The side effects listed in official booklets were daunting. Dr. Lewis and Dr. K. had said that this chemo would be easier than Barry's first chemo regimen we had had two years ago. But neither doctor could advise us about resuming work or other activities.

As it turned out, Barry didn't get nauseous; he felt well aside from some fatigue. He even started driving locally, and we took some slow walks around our neighborhood, did some shopping, and enjoyed the beautiful June weather.

On the Sunday after the treatment, Barry had an attack of vertigo. We were told this was "unrelated to the chemo," and it had occurred several weeks earlier as well. When he changed position quickly, he became suddenly dizzy, nauseous, and sweaty, and his skin became hot; very scary, whether you are having chemo or not. The first time it had happened, we hadn't known what to do, so we just waited it out. Barry just moved slowly for a day or two, and it subsided. This time, we reached for the Bonine, a medication for motion sickness that we had used on our boat trip in Alaska. It seemed to help, and within a few hours, Barry was able to rest more comfortably, gradually sitting up a little, and eating a tiny, light dinner. Why did these extra medical events pop up in the middle of cancer treatments? Two years ago, during his radiation therapy, there had been a bout of sciatica. And now, vertigo....... But all in all, we were both amazed at Barry's strength and his ability to tolerate this latest trial of chemo.

I found myself needing to nap again. After our week of being in emergency mode, I had to come down from it all. During the week of chemo, I had been happy to go to my physical exercise, but now I would have to rest and recover. Looking in the mirror told me what we had been through, and what I needed to do to get rid of the dark circles under my eyes.

We also had to consider our options for the coming week. Would Barry be able to see patients? People were being so understanding. But we wanted to give patients notice; you can't just book a day or a week of appointments overnight.

We decided to schedule patients, and give Barry Bonine early in the morning, in case the vertigo lingered. He would also move around slowly. On our way to the office, we stopped at the hospital for a shot of Nupagen to beef up his blood counts (which were devastated by the chemo) and to get some tests taken. We were hopeful about the new week, and happy Barry had tolerated the chemo so well.

Chapter Thirty-Eight

Another Problem

On the fourth day back at work, Barry moved slightly and felt pain like an electric jolt shoot up his spine. He thought he had pulled something in his back. He rested in his office for a minute and felt better. Back home, in the middle of the afternoon, it started to bother him again, and by six o'clock, he was having consistent sharp pains in his back. The pain came in bursts, causing him to grimace and arch his back and neck. It seemed to get worse every minute. This continued for over an hour. I found the pain pills I had left over from my root canal work. Barry took one and his pain eased remarkably.

With that relief we were able to go to sleep. In the middle of the night, I felt Barry jump. After seven hours, the stabbing jolts had returned. In thirty-six years of marriage, I had never seen my husband in such agony. He was sweating, grimacing, and every muscle in his back and neck tensed up each time he felt the shock. Now it seemed to be coming with his pulse. This was alarming; what could it be? Although he was a doctor, he was now the patient – I wondered: *Should I take him to the E.R. even though he didn't want me to?*

Barry decided to take another of my pain pills and try to rest. We knew that in the morning we were going to the hospital for his Nupagen shot and blood tests, and would see our local oncologist, Dr. R. We could consult with him. I didn't insist on calling an ambulance. When the pill took effect, the pain lessened. Barry's diagnosis was that this was a back spasm, caused by insult to the nerve. I guessed the other possibilities were meningitis, some sort of nerve damage, or something else too terrible to name.

In the morning, Barry got up gingerly, trying not to add insult to his injury. His back felt better, but the pain pill hadn't worn off yet; it would remain effective until a while after we saw the oncologist.

Dr. R. had to rule out any side effect of the chemo, and also something caused by the cancer itself. But after seeing the morning's blood tests, he was not alarmed. A pinched nerve could have this effect, and that must be what had happened. At least it was a temporary thing, and not something deadly. This we could handle.

After finishing at the hospital, we were slowly making our way across the street to our office when Barry's beeper went off. It was our secretary, and when we reached the office, she had an emergency patient for Barry to see. It seemed ridiculous for him to be in such bad shape, and still to be called about someone's eye problem. But it took our minds off his condition, and it allowed us to do something normal and productive - for a while.

We finally finished not only the week of chemo, but the week after, with its shots of Nupagen, blood tests and urinanalysis as well. We were past the worst. Barry's blood counts remained very low, so we had to continue the Nupagen for several more days, but that was a minor inconvenience. We had survived, and even done well, for the first treatment. We could handle this dreaded Ifosfamide!

One day that week, our secretary brought in a newspaper article. On closer examination, I saw that it was an obituary. One of our patients with cancer, a person who had been an inspiration to us, had finally succumbed to his disease, multiple myeloma. I found out later that he had been fighting it for over ten years. Here was a man who had been in our office a few months ago. Though he hadn't looked well, he was still working and enjoying life. His attitude had been astounding, something to strive for. And now he had lost his battle. I felt profound sadness. Later, it occurred to me that there was another way to look at it: he had gained ten years of life. But I didn't want Barry to hear this news just yet. Maybe I could keep it from him until we had some good news about his own situation to offset it.

CHAPTER THIRTY-NINE

A FEW WEEKS OFF

We now had three weeks off. No treatments, no shots, no medication, no doctors........normalcy. How we had once taken it for granted! As soon as Barry felt well again, we put all the medical issues behind us, and concentrated on these three wonderful weeks. They were filled with normal life: things that we had once hardly noticed, but now we savored.

Then a reminder: the hair loss...again. It started suddenly the second week after the chemo. Barry's hair fell out everywhere: onto his collar, on the floor, in the sink, you name it. Again Barry was self-conscious. He said he looked like a "frosted light bulb," that he didn't want to look "like a freak." I told our swimming buddies that he would be back at swimming soon, but was embarrassed about his baldness. One of our friends said, "Oh, good, now he'll look like me!"

At the office, we again began preparing the patients for the change in Barry's appearance. We had a few people coming in who had been in the previous week; what a shock for them to see how different their doctor looked in a matter of days. Then, of course, we had the handful who liked him without hair. One woman couldn't stop raving about what a gorgeous head he had, "Just like Yul Brynner!" Barry took out his collection of baseball hats. We had caps from Alaska and the Grand Canyon, and some in great colors like baby blue and "Rockport red" to match the lobster shack, "Motif #1", up on Cape Ann. In the past, I hadn't really cared for baseball caps; now, I loved them.

We were also expecting Sara and Richard to visit from Alaska. They arrived looking none the worse for their red-eye flight; they were young. As we drove home from the airport, it seemed so natural to have them with us. It was hard to believe that they lived halfway around the world, in such an inhospitable place. But they were adventurers and they loved their life in Fairbanks. Living in

Alaska had been a long-time dream of our son-in-law's; in their first apartment in Seattle, I had noticed a big map of Alaska on the wall.

The young couple brought us such a break from our medical worries. Their enthusiasm was contagious. The first time we had met Richard, when we were visiting our daughter in Seattle, we liked him immediately. Barry and I had been waiting at our motel for Sara and her boyfriend to meet us. As they approached, I stepped back to let Barry hug Sara; her boyfriend, Richard, astounded me by walking up to me with his arms outstretched, saying, with a big smile, "Hi! I'm Richard!" The young man's outgoing personality was one you just couldn't resist. Even Barry, the father who could be judgmental and critical, let down his reserve.

Now we packed so much into their four day visit with us. It had to be a short trip because both Sara and Richard had hectic schedules that summer. They were using the Fourth of July break to squeeze in a trip to New York. As wonderful as it was for us to see them, it was even better for them to see Barry, vital and energetic now despite his hair loss. They had been so worried about him.

We spent one day in New York City, wandering for hours in the Metropolitan Museum of Art, strolling down Fifth Avenue past all the famous stores, down to Rockefeller Center and into St. Patrick's Cathedral. After a brief rest there, we walked back uptown, stopping to browse in Tiffany's and then entered Central Park, past the boat basin, the Alice in Wonderland statue, and back to the museum where our car was parked. All these were things we had done many times before, but our son-in-law was from Los Angeles, and hadn't spent much time in New York, and he was enthralled. This made us see our home town through new eyes. We had wondered whether Barry could tolerate all this exercise, but he could, and, once again, he amazed us.

We spent a special day at my mother's home in New Jersey. What a treat for her to see Sara and Richard again. They were in touch frequently by mail and by phone, but you can't hug your granddaughter long-distance! We took lots of photos that day.

Though we were very active during their visit, we saved lots of time for just hanging around and talking. So many topics come up when you are lazing around, things that you don't get to talk about when you are busy all the time. It turned out to be a time that cemented our relationship and strengthened the love we all had for each other. When we took them to the airport for their return flight, Richard said he couldn't wait to visit again. That warmed our hearts.

CHAPTER FORTY

CYCLE 2 OF IFOSFAMIDE CHEMO
(July '01)

Within two days of Sara and Richard's departure, Barry and I were back in the hospital for his treatment. He was hooked up to his chemo and I was keeping vigil. It was cycle two of the heavy-duty drugs. Hard as it was, I was happy to have it underway. Each day that passed meant more medicine inside my husband's body, fighting his cancer. I was keeping my fingers crossed.

After the chemo was finished, I was wary, recalling the secondary problems that had developed after the past treatments: Barry's sciatica, the back and neck spasms, and the vertigo. Sure enough, the morning after the chemo, Barry woke up with a pain in his right shoulder, above and behind the spot where his port was. He thought he must have slept in a funny position, since he couldn't remember anything else that might have caused this pain.

During the day, we went out for a walk, but all the while, Barry was aware of the nagging pain in his shoulder. In the afternoon, it became more severe, and finally he was reduced to lying still with an ice pack on his shoulder. That, along with Tylenol, seemed to help. This was how we spent that weekend; he kept the pain at bay with ice and Tylenol.

The worry was as bad as the pain. Barry was concerned that the pain might be related to his mediport, or to vein damage from the chemo. We didn't know if this was muscle pain or something more serious. Again a problem had cropped up on the weekend, and we couldn't reach any of the oncologists for their opinions.

On Monday we returned to the hospital for the Nupagen shot and tests, and we were finally able to ask the chemo nurse about the shoulder pain. By then it was beginning to ease up, and, from our description, she said it was probably muscle pain. That was somewhat reassuring. She would mention it to the oncologist when she saw him, although by then we would be long gone and back working at our office. If the doctor was concerned about it, he would call us.

As the week progressed, the pain decreased, and Barry and I kept trying to figure out what on earth had caused it. Finally, I formulated my expert opinion: Barry had told me that he had done some push-ups during the chemo, while the drugs were flowing. How many, I asked him.................. the answer was 30! Thirty push-ups! During chemo! Now I thought I knew what had happened. When you get chemo, you get other drugs as well, including steroids. These suppress pain and inflammation. Barry had probably injured his shoulder, perhaps on the first, second, or even the tenth push-up; then, since the steroid masked the pain, he continued to do thirty repetitions. By the end, the injury was aggravated. Since Barry got the steroid throughout the week of the chemo, it wasn't until the day after the chemo that the steroids left his system and the pain kicked in.

Once we felt that Barry's injury wasn't serious, a lot of our stress was relieved. We still had to deal with the constant pain, which increased whenever Barry took a deep breath or coughed. But it gradually subsided and he could manage it.

CHAPTER FORTY-ONE

SIDE-EFFECTS

After two rounds of chemo, we had several weeks off before the next CAT scan and the subsequent treatment. We had to rest up, recover, and rebuild Barry's stamina, but we knew that that would come with time. One of the hard things about this chemo regimen was that as soon as he began to feel good, it would be time to get himself knocked down again. Submitting to poison. I just knew that in years to come, people would look back on this sort of treatment and consider it barbaric. But right now it was the only thing available to us, and we were grateful to be able to have it. Strange.

The week after the chemo, we were back at work, inching back into life. On Thursday night, when Barry got into bed, he said he felt something in his back. Something wasn't right. It wasn't pain - yet. He was worried, I could see. It was nighttime, so no medical people were be available, and after all the strange side-effects he had had in the past, we were wary.

As we lay in bed, trying to figure out what was happening, my mind was racing. Something rang a bell. Wasn't this the exact day in the last cycle when Barry's throbbing back pain had started? Could that be? I got out of bed and ran to read the chemo log I had been keeping throughout this course of treatment. Sure enough, there it was: on the Thursday of the week after chemo, Barry's back had started to give him pain. Last time we had thought it was some sort of injury, but this was too much of a coincidence. This had to be related to some part of his treatment.

Within minutes, the pain increased. It began as a pulse. Soon it was true pain, originating in his lower back and pulsing up his spine. Before long, the pain was severe, and, like last time, we resorted to taking one of the pain pills from my root canal work. The pill helped, but Barry had waited too long to take it. Pain like this has to be dealt with before it gets severe, or the medication isn't effective.

Finally, we put ice packs on his back, and that, with the medication, enabled him to sleep.

In the morning, we met the local oncologist at the hospital for blood tests, the urinanalysis and the Nupagen shot. Barry suspected that the pain in his bones was related to the Nupagen, which was supposed to stimulate his bone marrow to make more blood cells. He had been taking the Nupagen shots since the beginning of the week; why, then, did the pain start on the fourth day? Last month, the pain had lasted only 24 hours, even though he continued to get Nupagen for three more days. The oncologist didn't have the answer. He had patients who had had bone pain with Nupagen, but it wasn't severe, and had started shortly after getting the Nupagen shot, and lasted only until the shots were finished. Barry's pattern was not typical, if, in fact, this was the cause.

Later that day, we spoke to Dr. Lewis. As soon as Barry described his experience with the pulsing back pain, Dr. Lewis replied that it was a reaction to the Nupagen. He had seen it many times: the pain could be very severe; it could be pulsing; it could be in the bone marrow. It could last 24 hours, or frequently longer. What a relief it was to know the cause, and not to be worried that some other terrible thing was at the root of the pain. Barry had been afraid that the pain signified that his cancer had now spread to his bones. I know that he hadn't wanted to tell me this. Whatever the reason, Dr. Lewis again had saved us. This time, it was from our own worry. There was no way I could thank him enough.

You might think that as soon as the pain subsided, we were ready to celebrate. Not so. After days of severe pain, and the accompanying worry, Barry and I were drained, and in need of some "R and R." We had the weekend to recover, and we spent it resting. We needed to catch up on some real sleep. By Monday, we were able to return to work, and life, still somewhat dazed. It was astounding to me that we had gone through this experience, and nobody had warned us about this side-effect. I could only understand it by telling myself that this reaction must be rare, and that most oncologists hadn't seen it. In the forty years that I had known Barry, I had never seen him in such agony. I had felt caught between my own instinct to call 911 and my belief that I could best support Barry by not over-riding his own wishes.

CHAPTER FORTY-TWO

TIME OFF

Following our pattern of scheduling vacations just prior to CAT scans, we drove north to Ithaca for a short but very welcome mini-vacation. The leisurely pace of life in upstate New York was restorative. We saw generations of families enjoying picnics together at the lake, spreading tablecloths on the wooden tables, unpacking mountains of food. Many were taking walks along the trails in the park. Some guided small motor boats out onto Lake Cayuga, with all the kids safely in their life preservers, and spent the sunny summer day floating around on the blue, blue waters surrounded by rolling green hills. Then there were the teenagers, zooming in their motorboats or jet-ski's across the water, making as much noise as they could. We loved eating lunch at the snack bar near the lake. We ate hot dogs and French fries, so different from what we allowed ourselves at home since we were always watching our fat intake..... It was the taste of another life.

Somehow, we had learned to put unpleasant things out of our minds, or at least to the side. This enabled us to enjoy our time off without dwelling on the looming CAT scan. People with serious illnesses learn to deal with situations in ways they never could have imagined. In the past I had looked at people with cancer and wondered how they could smile, laugh, or enjoy anything. Now I understood it and felt it, without knowing how we developed the strength.

CHAPTER FORTY-THREE

BACK TO REALITY
(Aug '01)

Back home, the Monday morning of the CAT scan arrived and our nervousness returned. The chemo that Barry had just been taking was the most potent chemotherapy regimen available for his kind of cancer at this stage. We were anxious to learn the results of the treatment. Somehow we remained outwardly calm. Along with our fears, we had hopes that this drug would work.

After the scan, we were back at our office seeing patients, when I called the hospital to be sure they had faxed the report to our doctors: Dr. Lewis, of course, Dr. K., the oncologist at Sloan-Kettering, and Dr. R., our local oncologist. To my surprise, the person on the other end of the phone offered to fax me the report as well. I agreed; I wanted to read it for myself. Within minutes, our fax machine was buzzing and I held the report in my hands.

The first thing I read was that my husband's lungs were clear. My heart leaped, but there was more. I held my breath and read on. The second paragraph stated that the tumor in his liver had grown. Grown while on this heavy duty chemo! There were also several new, smaller tumors scattered throughout his liver. More cancer, while undergoing treatment? I felt devastated. I didn't understand how this could be happening.

Apparently, the sarcoma metastases in Barry's lungs were susceptible to chemo, but those in his liver were not. None of the doctors could account for this. Was this difference in the tumors themselves or in the blood supply which delivered the drug to those organs? Nobody knew. And nobody knew what to do next.

I Fed-Exed the CAT scan to Dr. K., our oncologist at Sloan-Kettering; we had an appointment with him that Friday, and we wanted him to have the films in advance. But when we arrived at our appointment four days later, neither he nor his staff had looked at the scans. In fact, they had trouble locating them. We tried to remain calm. Dr. K. outlined our two remaining options: surgery or embolization of the large tumor, followed by a different chemo to deal with the smaller tumors. Barry had already had the best and most promising drugs. He wondered how effective the one remaining drug could be. Dr. K. told us he would present the case to the "Liver Committee" at Sloan-Kettering, and give us their advice. We left for home, grim and losing hope.

When we consulted with Dr. Lewis, he told us not to give up. He had seen large tumors embolized, which seemed to have a beneficial effect on the smaller tumors. He couldn't account for it or explain the mechanism, but it had happened. He made us feel that there was still reason to hope.

We called Dr. B., the leading authority on sarcoma. He was about to leave on vacation, but he did call us back. My husband spoke to him briefly. I watched and waited. Barry was not smiling. Dr. B. was not the cheerleader that Dr. Lewis was.

Finally, Dr. K. called us with his suggestion: the Liver Committee had recommended surgery, and a liver surgeon, Dr. D. would see us in two days if we would call him immediately. We called even though Barry dreaded the thought of liver surgery. It would be complicated, since the tumor was very high on the dome of the liver, just underneath the lungs. And Barry didn't want to go through such an ordeal just to have to deal with numerous smaller tumors afterwards.

With fear in our hearts, and dread in our bones, the two of us made our way to Sloan-Kettering, to meet a new surgeon. At least we had each other, and whatever time we had left.

CHAPTER FORTY-FOUR

EMBOLIZATION

We met with the Liver Surgeon, Dr. D., on a Thursday morning. He seemed to be a caring and competent person. Given all the details of Barry's situation, Dr. D. did not recommend surgery. He suggested embolization instead, which was a procedure to cut off the blood supply to the tumor. The embolization would be performed by an invasive radiologist at Sloan, but Dr. D. himself would admit my husband to the surgery floor of the hospital, order the procedure, and oversee Barry's hospitalization until he was stable. After a few weeks of recuperation, a new chemo regimen would begin.

There were several potential complications of the embolization, some of them serious. Dr. D. spoke especially about the risks of infection and puncturing the lungs. After the tumor's blood supply was cut off, the tumor itself would die, and the patient's body would have to clean it up. We listened to the details with mounting fear, as determined as we were to face this with courage and dignity. Our next hurdle was to get on the schedule. Sloan-Kettering was very busy and at first we were told that we would have to wait a month for the procedure. In the meantime, we were put on a waiting list and Barry began the pre-admission testing.

Dr. Lewis told us that the embolization would be "a piece of cake" after what we had been through. This was hard to believe, but it helped to hear some positive talk in the face of all the pessimism. He also suggested that we go on a vacation. We didn't know how or when we could, but we did start thinking about trying. I wondered if he was telling us that it was now or never, but I shied away from that train of thought.

A week after our meeting with Dr. D., his nurse called us on a Friday to say there was a cancellation the following Monday. Could Barry come in for the procedure then? We leapt into action. We had the weekend to get our medical papers ready, pay bills that needed to be paid the following week, get coverage for our office practice, and prepare ourselves mentally for the embolization procedure. I remembered Barry's first hospitalization and surgery, three years earlier, and all the arrangements I had to make. This time I knew better what to expect. I prepared to be away from our office for several days and for daily trips to and from Sloan-Kettering. I found all the important forms we needed for the hospital, and I called our family members to let them know the plan.

We were to register at Sloan-Kettering at 7AM on Monday. This meant leaving our house at 5:30, and driving down to the city in the dark. How many times had we done this now? It was getting to be routine, and, oddly enough, there was something beautiful and calming about the quiet, early morning trip.

The admissions office at Sloan-Kettering is very efficient. The patient and his family are processed through the various rooms leading up to the Pre-Surgery Center. There patients change into hospital garb, get hooked up to their IV's, and wait to be called for their procedures. It is humbling to be a part of the variety of humanity there; people of all ages, colors, nationalities - all trying desperately to save their lives. Every patient has a caring family member or friend wheeling him around, listening to the doctors and nurses, and trying to be brave.

When Barry was called for the embolization, I was able to go with him as far as the procedure room. A young radiologist explained what she was planning to do, but I noticed that she used the word "if" a lot. She did not take it for granted that she would be able to do everything she hoped to do. She was going to thread a catheter up an artery in Barry's leg, and when it reached the point where it delivered blood to the tumor in the liver, she would send up pellets of some sort to block the blood supply. This would cause the tumor to die. The trick was to do this without doing too much damage to the liver itself. I guessed this depended on exactly where the blood vessels went and whether she could cut off the blood supply to the tumor without compromising the liver.

Then the radiologist asked us about the latest CAT scan. It had not been digitized into the Sloan-Kettering system yet. *How could that be?* This was the scan that I had Fed-Exed to our Sloan-Kettering oncologist three weeks earlier, the one that the surgeon, Dr. D. had had trouble locating when we met him. How could this venerated institution slip up so often? I was alarmed because the missing scan was the latest picture of the tumor. But the radiologist did not seem concerned. She said she could look at Barry's liver in "real time" while doing the embolization.

When the radiologist was ready to begin, I left the procedure room, with an hour to myself before checking back with them. Though I had several offers from Ellen and from friends to wait with me during the procedure, I had declined them all. I wanted time alone. And nobody else would have been permitted to go up to the Pre-Surgery Center. I didn't want to have anyone waiting downstairs for me while I was with Barry. I didn't want to be worrying about anyone else that day.

I made my way through the lobby of the hospital to the cafeteria. I wanted comfort food. All I could eat those days was chocolate, so a large chocolate chip cookie and a cup of hot chocolate were in order. On the way back, I stopped at the telephone bank in the lobby to call our insurance company for the umpteenth time. We were still trying to get approval for this procedure. Both Dr. D.'s office and I had called them in advance of the embolization to get it pre-certified, but we had not been successful. After numerous phone calls, approval was still not forthcoming, and now the insurance company was requesting more information. I even went so far as to leave an emotional message for a supervisor at the company about this procedure saving my husband's life, and that we had called long in advance for this approval, and that I was not going to jeopardize his care by delaying the embolization while they played their games. It probably did no good, but it helped me vent. This was just one of many calls I was to make to the insurance company in the coming weeks, where I let out my feelings on the phone and then calmed down for the rest of the world.

When I returned to the area outside the procedure room, a nurse told me that Barry would be out in a few minutes. *So soon? Did this mean that they hadn't been able to complete it?* My heart was pounding, but they told me that it had gone well, and they were finishing up.

Before we knew it, Barry and I were back in the Pre-Surgery Center, where we would stay until he had stabilized. He was alert and his color had returned, though he was still heavily medicated. I called Ellen, telling her she could come to the hospital and meet us upstairs as soon as we had been assigned a hospital room for his stay. I took a deep breath. The embolization was over.

For twenty-four hours after the procedure, Barry was on a morphine drip for severe pain. But by the afternoon following the embolization, he wasn't using it at all and the drip was disconnected. He looked great, and felt great. Once again, his outward appearance belied what was happening inside. We were now on the lookout for fever, one of the after-effects of the procedure which could signal either infection or just the body's dealing with the dying tumor.

Barry was in the hospital for three days, and I drove down each morning and home each night, taking my daughter home with me the first night. It was great to have Ellen's company. When we returned to the city the next morning, we decided to take the train instead of driving, and to walk uptown from Grand Central Station to Sloan-Kettering. While I was visiting Barry at the hospital, I wasn't getting any of my regular exercise, so the walk would do me good. I must admit, it was fun to walk with Ellen through the early morning streets of Manhattan. We walked at a good pace, and by the time we reached 68th Street, I was sweating.

After three days in the hospital, the doctors were ready to discharge Barry. The night before his release, the surgeon and his team made rounds, and said that Barry looked ready to go home, although they were reluctant to let him leave too early. Most patients develop a fever, and they didn't want to send Barry home only to have the fever occur later. Nevertheless, he was doing so well that they decided to let him go.

CHAPTER FORTY-FIVE

RETURN TO SLOAN

At home, we monitored Barry's temperature. Sure enough, our first night at home, a fever developed, then it rose to the point at which we were supposed to report it. It was evening, so we spoke to the on-call doctor, who told us to call the surgeon's office in the morning. The following day, the fever had risen higher, and the surgeon's nurse said we needed to return to Sloan. By then it was Friday afternoon. Once again, we jumped into the car, and sped down to the city. It was rush hour, and traffic was awful. I was trying my best to get my sick husband to the hospital. Barry said he felt like I was a NASCAR driver! (That was a compliment.)

We arrived at Sloan-Kettering's "Urgent Care Center," their Emergency Room, late on Friday. It was packed. You would have thought they were giving something away. Everyone there was a Sloan patient with some sort of emergency. There wasn't enough room, and the nurses and doctors were working feverishly. In the cubicle next to Barry's, we heard a neurologist questioning a patient: did the man know what day it was; what year it was? They suspected that he had had a stroke. Barry and I looked at each other and laughed in spite of ourselves; did we even know what day it was? I don't think so.

When Barry was examined, he was admitted to the hospital, but there were no beds available upstairs. There were ten or fifteen patients in the same situation, waiting on stretchers. The nurses had to clear out the emergency area because new patients were arriving continuously, so they put those awaiting hospital beds in an adjacent area used for clinics during the day. Meanwhile, it was growing late. It was too late for me to go all the way home, and I wanted to stay with Barry until he was placed in a hospital room, so I decided to stay overnight.

As unbelievable as it sounds, my husband was "settled" with pillow and blankets, along with his IV pole and apparatus, on a couch in the clinic waiting room. This was to be his bed for the night, since no beds were expected to open up in regular hospital rooms. I lay down next to his couch on two chairs pushed together. When the Emergency Room was finally cleared out at 1 A.M., the staff moved Barry back to that area to sleep on a stretcher. I took his place on the couch in the waiting room nearby. All night long, I watched hospital security guards make their rounds through this supposedly unused portion of the facility.

It wasn't until the following afternoon that a bed opened up and Barry was moved upstairs to a hospital room. It was hard to believe how busy Sloan was. By now, some of Barry's blood tests had come back, and luckily, they showed no infection. The doctor had been worried about an abscess forming as the large tumor died. I know that Barry had been worrying about this as well. So far, it seemed that he would avoid that complication.

Barry spent four more days in the hospital. Though he felt better each day, he still ran fevers and was given strong antibiotics. Ellen and I saw him daily, but he didn't feel up to having any other visitors.

Barry was in a semi-private room, and his roommate was a priest from Italy with minimal knowledge of English. Barry ordered the priest's food for him, since he just couldn't make himself understood to the staff. This provided some comic relief, since the man had trouble communicating with everyone from the doctors and nurses right down to the food-service personnel. At one point, when the doctors had been unable to perform a procedure on him because of a heart problem, the priest was wheeled back into the room, with nine medical people working on him to stabilize his heart. It happened that all of these doctors and nurses were women. Since he had been complaining earlier that he was being "neglected," the surgical resident asked him if he felt important now with so many people working on him. He replied, "I am priest. Women cannot make me feel important." We overheard this conversation from behind the curtain in our half of the room. Our mouths dropped open. In the eyes of this priest, these dedicated doctors, nurses and technicians were not medical people, they were merely women.

Each day that Barry was in the hospital, he received at least one phone call from Dr. Lewis. This was comforting in the midst of so much uncertainty and fear. Meanwhile, I was still making my own phone calls to our insurance company, pursuing approval for the original embolization procedure. It got to the point where the pre-certification person recognized my voice without me even saying my name. They were still working on it. It had been rejected once, and was in appeal. Later, they would reject it for a second time, and it would go into their second appeal. This went on and on. It was discouraging and worrisome, but it made me determined to do something about this type of situation when the dust cleared. It was just not right for people dealing with severe medical problems to have to fight for their insurance coverage. In the United States we are proud to have the most advanced medical care in the world, yet we have an inhumane system of medical insurance, where business people (rather than medical people) decide which patients are allowed to have which care. Is this crazy or what? And what about all the patients who are too sick or too old to argue with their insurance carriers? I call this unconscionable.

CHAPTER FORTY-SIX

HOME AGAIN
(Sept – Oct '01)

O ur daughter Ellen continued to visit the hospital and provide support. She would be leaving the area soon, spending several weeks working with theatre groups outside the city, as part of a grant she had received. Luckily, her schedule allowed her to visit us in the hospital while Barry was still an inpatient. When she left the city to pursue her work, he was discharged from the hospital.

When I went to pick Barry up at Sloan-Kettering, I encountered a long line of traffic waiting to get into the hospital parking garage. I waited in the line for ten or fifteen minutes, and was still not inside the garage. I had never seen so many people trying to get into Sloan's garage at one time. As I was approaching the entrance to the garage, I called Barry in his hospital room to tell him that I would be there soon. He answered that the doctor had discharged him already, and he was waiting for me. He felt good and wanted to come downstairs himself. He told me to drive around to the front of the building and meet him. I couldn't believe it, but I agreed. I carefully maneuvered my Jeep out of the line-up, drove around the block, and stopped at Sloan-Kettering's front door. Barry walked out and got in the car, and the hospitalization was over!

It was great to be home again, and to do regular things. We took the days slowly, but tried to get out and around as Barry recuperated. He would remain on antibiotics for another week to prevent any infections from occurring. But as the days passed, Barry developed a severe cough that seemed to cause more trouble than the procedure itself. He agreed to call a colleague, Dr. E., an ear, nose, and throat specialist whom we had known for many years. Of course, Dr. E. said to come right to his office. He suspected the cough was a side effect of the antibiotic. Dr. E. examined Barry and gave him some medication that brought him considerable relief. Barry had been coughing for days. His throat was raspy, and his stomach muscles were sore. Who knew that this could be caused by an antibiotic? I knew that Barry had been afraid that his tumor was the cause, and that it was growing and irritating his diaphragm. Now that we knew the source of the problem, his concern lessened. The cough gradually resolved, but, as the doctor had warned us, it remained for several weeks after the last dose of the antibiotic.

All during this time, I continued to call our insurance company to get authorization for the embolization procedure. I had submitted a lot of information, and they had also obtained hospital records and documentation from the surgeon. Still, approval was not forthcoming.

Barry mentioned the trouble we were having with the insurance company to Dr. Lewis in one of their conversations. Without hesitation, Dr. Lewis asked if there was anything he could do. Barry didn't know whether or not it would help, but since Dr. Lewis was a world specialist in sarcoma, a note from him might influence our insurance company. Dr. Lewis thought a phone call would be more effective. If we would get him the name and phone number of the medical director of the insurance company, he would be glad to call him.

Early the next morning, I called the pre-cert person at our insurance company for the name and phone number of their medical director. Without wasting time, I gave the information to Dr. Lewis's secretary. You can imagine my surprise when, in about an hour, Dr. Lewis's secretary returned my call, telling me she had a message for me from Dr. Lewis: he had spoken with the medical director, and expected the situation to be cleared up soon. I couldn't believe my ears. *How could Dr. Lewis have managed this with one phone call?* I was speechless. I only managed to murmur my thanks to the secretary.

Dr. Lewis's help relieved some of my anxiety about the financial burden of this procedure. I knew that there was no question about having it done, and even if another embolization became necessary, there was no doubt that we would do that as well. We would find a way. But it was a great help that our insurance would cover a portion of it. Now all we had to do was to wait for the insurance company to

complete their deliberations.....and it did happen. Three weeks after
Dr. Lewis's phone call, we got word that the embolization had been
approved by the committee.

Within a week after the hospital discharge, we were back
working in Barry's office seeing patients. We liked returning to the
structure of a schedule. But we were beginning to feel that Barry
should consider retiring. We had been battling this cancer for three
and a half years and we were tired. Running the practice was a lot
of responsibility on top of our own medical worries. This issue
played on our minds, and every now and then we would discuss it. I
think that Barry felt that he had had enough of fixing other people's
problems. His own were becoming too much of a burden. I agreed,
although I feared that without the practice we would have nothing to
focus on except his illness.

CHAPTER FORTY-SEVEN

TERRORISM & CHEMO

It was a Tuesday morning, we were working in the office, and we were scheduled to start the new chemo the following day. It was Sept. 11, 2001. We, along with every other New Yorker, along with every other American, experienced the unspeakable horror of the attacks on the World Trade Center and the Pentagon.

Everyone who lived through that day knows the shock and fear of those attacks: the evil and hatred of the terrorists, the bravery of the victims and the rescue workers. For me, it was too much to comprehend. I was trying to deal with cancer and its recurrence, and didn't know how to add another horror to my experience.

So I focused on the here and now: the daily things I had to do. Make sure my family was safe; pay the bills; drive Barry to chemo; send money to the Red Cross; watch the news for latest updates; check the office messages. The daily trivia blended with the extraordinary; one minute you were buying milk, and the next you were trying to donate blood. They had enough blood - just send money. Then watching the news video of the rescue workers, ready to sacrifice everything. Then watching the poison chemo dripping down the IV line into Barry's weary body. It was surreal - but not just for me and my husband - for everyone I knew, and for those I didn't know. There are no words to express the feelings of those days. We just went on, minute by minute, day by day, trying to do the right thing and to keep life in perspective. I felt keenly that here we were, trying to make use of the newest medical advances, trying to save Barry's life, while a few days ago, thousands of healthy Americans had had their lives snuffed out instantaneously. A moment of terror. A flash. Who could make sense of such insanity?

Barry received his new chemo treatments, and seemed to do pretty well. The most debilitating side-effects were weakness and tiredness. These increased with each weekly dose, so that by the fourth and last one, he was wiped out. He was able to work on the days between doses, and since he got the chemo at our local hospital, it was as convenient as chemo can be.

Somewhere in those weeks, the true horror of the terrorist attacks hit me, and for several days, I cried and was jumpy all the time. I knew many people who were experiencing this kind of thing; there was a delay between the traumatic occurrence and its integration into our minds. Afterwards, it seemed to hit me in waves every few days. I couldn't imagine how people who had lost loved ones were coping.

Barry and I had several days off between the last chemo treatment and his next CAT scan, so we decided get away to Ithaca. We were lucky to get a motel reservation on fairly short notice. Someone asked me if we would be visiting anyone up in Ithaca. "We're revisiting our youth," I replied. It was the truth.

I did the driving this time, and we sailed through the New York suburbs and farmland, past rolling hills with magnificent fall color. We turned the car radio on and learned of the start of the United States' retaliatory bombing of Afghanistan. Chills ran through my body. We expected this, but still it was frightening. Would this make the terrorists step up their activities and strike again, as they had threatened?

So many conflicting emotions were running through my heart and mind. Barry and I were on the way to a relaxing vacation. The countryside was beautiful: fall in its splendor. We were about to celebrate our 36th anniversary, which we had thought we'd never see. At the same time, we were also still reeling from the shock of the terrorist strike on our country, and the sadness of all the lives cut short, all the children now orphans. And now we were fearful about our country's bombing strikes in the Middle East. Not to mention our own looming CAT scan. What a vacation. How on earth could anyone relax while dragging along such baggage? All I can say is, we tried our best.

When we checked in to our motel, we found flowers waiting for us: our children had sent them for our anniversary. I felt like a celebrity.

We spent four days driving around Ithaca, stopping at our favorite places. Barry's energy level was extremely low, so hiking and even walking any distance was out of the question. We took a lot of naps. We also were glued to the television news coverage, showing our fighter planes on the other side of the globe, and the threats to Americans broadcast from Osama Bin Laden's headquarters, some hidden place in the Afghan mountains. We celebrated our anniversary at a restaurant we had each been to on our first nights in college. It was a custom of dorm counselors to take their new freshman charges to "Joe's." We loved this old-fashioned restaurant; it was in "downtown" Ithaca, and served delicious Italian dishes.

The state parks were not crowded since it was well after the summer season, and we had them mostly to ourselves. At one of our favorite spots, we saw a blue heron swoop down near a waterfall and wade in a stream. It was magical! Squirrels dropped acorns on us from trees high above.

One day, we were at a rocky viewpoint in a park, enjoying the view of a distant waterfall. It was during the school year, and several students were nearby. As we were starting to climb the rock steps back to the parking lot, Barry stumbled and fell. The students rushed over to help him, offering to assist him the entire way. He thanked them and declined, but we were sobered. We were face to face with Barry's deteriorating stamina, his loss of balance. When I looked at him now, I saw an aging man, no longer confident in his physical ability. How different he was from even a few months ago.

When you are engaged in a battle with cancer, it is hard to describe your frustration and fear. You cannot see your enemy, you do not know its tactics, where it will strike next, what it will be susceptible to, what it will shrug off. You can enlist the best experts, but with some forms of cancer, there is simply nobody who knows what will be effective. Dedicated people have been researching treatments for years, and there is so much they still just don't know. Dr. Lewis had described his own frustration at how long it took to do experimental trials with each individual drug agent you hope will prove effective. So you fight your war, using every conceivable weapon, but you are fighting blindfolded, totally in the dark, against a formidable, insidious adversary who strikes guerilla-style, showing no mercy.

CHAPTER FORTY-EIGHT

UNCHARTED COURSE

As soon as Barry was home and completed his CAT scan, we were in a frenzy of activity. The scramble to obtain the initial reading; the opinions of the experts; support from our guardian angel, Dr. Lewis. This time, the local radiologist who read the scan did not write a detailed report; the reading was short. It showed "marked progression" of the cancer. What did that mean? Were there more tumors? Were the old ones growing? And what about the one that had been embolized? Barry was despondent, said it didn't matter - whatever it was, it was.

We were to see the liver surgeon, Dr. D. in a few days, but Dr. Lewis advised an appointment with Dr. K., the Sloan oncologist, as well. Dr. Lewis had already spoken to Dr. K., and they had agreed on yet another course of treatment. All the doctors offered their clinical expertise, but Dr. Lewis was the only one who encouraged us, who told us what he would do, who cared enough to ask how we were doing emotionally, who seemed to want Barry to survive.

The sarcoma was on the move - growing and spreading in my husband's liver. Here was a man who looked so healthy, who felt so good, yet cancer was eating him alive. And my frustration was that in a few years, modern medicine might have a cure for it. Could we keep Barry alive long enough? I knew so many people who died just a little too soon.

We went to Sloan-Kettering two days in a row, to see the liver surgeon and then the oncologist. On the first day, on our way to the doctor's appointment, we met our daughter for breakfast. Ellen was hard at work on a project for another grant she had received, and was working at Lincoln Center with a famous director. It was wonderful to see her so happy. When you are in the middle of serious medical treatment, it is so good to have something else to focus on, to have some good news in your life.

As we left Ellen and walked to Sloan, we returned to the dark world of cancer. We met with the surgeon, Dr. D., who was kind but somber, and had the sad job of telling us the bad news. The big tumor, which had been embolized, was only half-dead. The doctor said this was still considered fairly successful, and further embolizations were possible, but what we needed more than that right now was a drug that would deal with the many other tumors which were growing in size and multiplying in number. There were no effective drug agents left to deal with sarcoma; Barry had tried all the available and known chemical treatments. None of them had been effective in his liver, although they had eliminated the tumors in his lungs. Dr. D. didn't understand why, and neither did anyone else. Meanwhile, he recommended the same treatment that Dr. K. and Dr. Lewis had agreed upon: Thalidomide, a drug which had been used to block the growth of new blood vessels to tumors in other forms of cancer. We had exhausted all the regimens known to work on sarcoma. After more than three and a half years of treatment, we were left to grasp at straws.

The next morning, we met with Dr. K., the oncologist who had prescribed all the chemo for Barry in the past. He was the renowned expert on sarcoma chemotherapy, and he had given us his best shots already. But he did not say there was nothing left; he, too, wanted us to try Thalidomide. He also told us that he had heard of a study being done on sarcoma patients at M. D. Anderson Cancer Center in Houston, Texas. Before we left, he gave us the phone number of M. D. Anderson, but we agreed to try the Thalidomide first. I could tell that Dr. K. was trying to be supportive, though was not much positive to say. However, I appreciated his efforts. This was the man who had tried to dash our hopes on the first day we had met him. The one I had cursed for being so pessimistic and assuming that we had no chance of winning the battle. Now Barry said that Dr. K. had known what he was talking about all along: once sarcoma goes to the liver, the game is over. I rejected that. Even if it were true, there was no reason for a doctor to take away a patient's hope.

All during this week, Barry felt tired, weak and achy, and we didn't know whether he was reacting to a recent flu-shot or to the cancer. We now knew that it would just be a question of time before he started feeling like a cancer patient again. But still I had a glimmer of hope that the Thalidomide would work.

As soon as we got home, Barry asked me to call M. D. Anderson Cancer Center in Texas. That encouraged me - not because I expected a miracle, but because it showed me that Barry still wanted to try. However, the person reviewing the experimental trials told us that she wasn't aware of any sarcoma studies that sounded like the one mentioned by Dr. K. She told us to check their web site, which I intended to do.

After the medical appointments of the week, we called Dr. Lewis late on Friday to check in. He tried to lift our spirits and told us that he had seen clinical evidence of patients who had not responded to chemotherapy, who had nevertheless tried Thalidomide and had their tumors stopped in their tracks. We did not ask if these were sarcoma patients; we didn't want to know. We did know by now that our odds were diminishing, yet we wanted some hope to cling to. Dr. Lewis agreed with Barry that traveling to M. D. Anderson Hospital in Texas to participate in a study that no one knew would be effective was not productive, and not a good way to use Barry's time, especially if that time was limited.

About a week earlier Barry had asked Dr. Lewis, "How long do you think I'll live?" The doctor had replied that he didn't know. This was a change from the unequivocal optimism of the past. But I trusted Dr. Lewis to tell us the truth, not necessarily to tell the whole truth, but at least the part we had asked for. He could tell from the question how much we wanted to know, how much we could handle. He was exquisitely sensitive to a patient's state of mind. He believed in being truthful, yet he knew that offering too much "truth" when the patient wasn't prepared to handle it, was cruel.

We were in a new stage now, one of just trying to stay alive. We had already given up hope of curing this awful disease, and had just been trying to keep the sarcoma from progressing. But now we had gone a little further down, lost a little more hope. There was one last shred to cling to: that Thalidomide would stop the tumors from growing new blood vessels. Since Thalidomide worked in a different way from the drugs we had tried, perhaps the tumors would respond. But this time, I felt that it was a long shot. I know Barry did, too. He said to me quietly one day, "I didn't think it would be such a short ride."

CHAPTER FORTY-NINE

THALIDOMIDE

With the prescription for Thalidomide in our hands, we drove directly to our local pharmacy with hopes of picking up the new drug. Not so fast: Thalidomide was a tightly controlled substance; pharmacies were not allowed to stock it. It had to be ordered and delivered for a specific patient, and this could happen only after Barry had filled out papers and received an authorization number from the manufacturer, and the pharmacy itself had received approval. These precautions were in place because decades earlier, when Thalidomide had been used to relieve morning sickness in pregnant women, it had caused birth defects in their babies.

Within a week we received the drug. Barry was to take four pills each night at home. That was it. No IV's, no pain, no hospital visits. After four weeks, we would see the Sloan-Kettering oncologist, who would check Barry out and give us the next month's prescription. This drug was regulated carefully and the manufacturer released only one month's supply at a time. We were grateful that there were no terrible side-effects of the Thalidomide. Barry felt tired and a little dizzy in the mornings, but he was able to function and he felt physically comfortable. Thus began our new regimen.

Meanwhile, fall had come and the colors were brilliant all around us. Every day we drove through magnificent country scenery, back and forth to our office and to town, and marveled at our luck to live in such a beautiful place. It always struck me that such natural beauty was fleeting; only as breathtaking as it was short-lived.

The contrasts in my mind were dizzying: outside, the world was aflame, nature was in her glory. Inside, Barry and I were waging a life and death battle with an invisible opponent. And nobody knew how to win this battle. It's one thing when you know what to do, even if it's hard; then you know that if you can get through it, it will be okay. But when the experienced specialists are only guessing, it's terrifying. I know that Barry believed that there was no hope left. He was trying this last drug because he wasn't ready to give up, but he felt that his days were numbered. I wasn't able to face this scenario.

With all of this fear in our minds, we continued to weigh the pros and cons of retiring from Barry's medical practice. It was a miracle that he had been able to keep on working for the past three and a half years through his cancer treatment. And, as sick as he was, he still felt able to see patients in his office. If any of his treatments worked, there was no reason to retire yet. And work took our minds off the disease.

Often, when I was at the office, patients would call up and ask to speak to me, just wondering how Barry was doing and to send their regards. Many people were praying for him every night. These people were more than patients - they cared about us and we cared about them. It was heartening to receive their concern. It made me feel less alone.

Retiring is a big step. Closing a practice is a major decision that cannot be undone. I knew that eventually we would have to deal with our employees, the office equipment and furniture, and the office lease, and, most importantly, transferring the patient records to another doctor. Physically, mentally, and emotionally, this was a weighty challenge that had to be tackled. I felt that the time had come.

While all this was happening, Barry continued with medication to control the spasmic cough that had started after the embolization. We thought the cough was getting better, but progress was slow. Gradually, however, we noticed other changes. Barry developed a cold, followed by a week or more of weakness, tiredness, new coughing, pain in his side when he took deep breaths, and, finally, shortness of breath. Barry assumed these symptoms were due to the cancer's progression. But one afternoon when we were talking to Dr. Lewis, he told us that if these symptoms persisted we should consult our local oncologist to rule out pneumonia. Later in the day, when Barry felt worse, he called the local doctor. We arranged to see him the following morning.

That next day, Saturday, was a long one for us. The doctor didn't like the way Barry's lungs sounded. He ordered a chest x-ray, which proved inconclusive, and didn't reveal any pneumonia. Now the oncologist wanted Barry to have a CAT scan, to rule out pulmonary emboli. These could be caused by Thalidomide, although usually only when it was combined with chemo and after prolonged use. Nevertheless, we had to be cautious because 'P.E.' could be deadly. I was alarmed. Barry thought that having a P.E. would not be "a bad way to go."

We drove to the local hospital and prepared for the CAT scan. Thank goodness the radiology department was staffed on the week-ends. After the scan, the reading by the radiologist, and the conference between the radiologist and the oncologist, we got the phone call telling us that there were no pulmonary emboli. I cannot describe my feelings of relief; we had good news for a change. I was only too happy to pick up the antibiotic for my husband. Whatever the problem, this would take care of it. The relief brought exhaustion for me, but Barry had once again been given a steroid at the hospital, and was flying-high. He couldn't sit still, while I was prone on the couch. This always happened when he took a steroid, and it made us laugh, once again. We still had our sense of humor! We even went out for pizza that night.

CHAPTER FIFTY

PNEUMONIA
(Nov '01)

We spent a quiet weekend as Barry recovered from his lung problems. The weather was glorious - beautiful, crisp, sunny fall days. It was a pleasure to be alive in this season, though we couldn't take walks or even be outside in it right now.

On Monday morning we had an appointment with Dr. Lewis in New York City, which we wouldn't have missed for the world. We were going to meet Ellen for lunch afterwards.

The early morning air was chilly, and Barry's breathing was labored, but we took the train into the city and slowly made our way walking from Grand Central Station to Dr. Lewis's office. On the way, we passed St. Patrick's Church on Fifth Avenue. The avenue itself was blocked off by fire trucks. There was a double funeral going on for two fallen firefighters, men who had been heroes in the Sept.11 attacks. Swarms of onlookers surrounded many, many uniformed firemen, all there to honor their brothers. Two fire trucks were parked back to back along Fifth Avenue, with their ladders fully extended, and uniformed men stood at attention up high in the raised buckets, saluting their fallen comrades. The sight was breathtaking. A lot of the onlookers had tears in their eyes. I did, too.

Our visit with Dr. Lewis was great for the soul, as usual. He was happy to see how good Barry looked. He said that if he saw my husband walking down the street, he would not suspect that he had cancer. Then he repeated his promise to be there for us as the disease took its toll. We were not alone. This compassionate and capable man would help us through whatever came next. He told us to call him at the end of the week. In addition, when I asked about a vacation, he encouraged us to take one. He believed in celebrating life, and was not afraid to live it, in spite of the fearful mood in the city since the recent attacks. Looking back on that visit now, I don't know what I was thinking. How could I consider a vacation with

Barry in the condition he was in? Yet, Dr. Lewis must have felt that if I asked this, why discourage us?

I left the meeting feeling buoyed by Dr. Lewis's enthusiasm for life, and his kindness to us. Then we turned our attention to our daughter, who was waiting for us. The three of us sat and talked over lunch, taking our time to enjoy each other. Ellen had chosen the theatre, an impossibly difficult field. But she was having success and she loved the work. She sure had guts to risk everything for this career. As protective as we were, we admired her for it. What more does a parent want?

As the three of us walked the few blocks towards the indoor passage to Grand Central Station, Barry began to have trouble breathing. He was freezing. That was strange; I was usually the cold one. I realized that he wasn't feeling well at all, and we walked very slowly. He refused to call a cab; he still needed to feel he could walk. I didn't want to insist, which would convey the message, *"You can't make it."* Once at Grand Central, we were able to rest before boarding our train home. Finally, we said good-bye to Ellen, found the gate for our train, and were able to relax while the train sped northward.

As it turned out, Barry did develop pneumonia, and bronchitis, as well. We ended up canceling all his office appointments for the week, and he spent the time resting. He was running fevers, and the local doctor put him on an antibiotic, as well as inhalers for the asthma that accompanied the pneumonia. For someone who had never taken any medication in his life, Barry was on an unbelievable number of drugs now. And then on other drugs to counteract the side-effects of these drugs. We had been so lucky before; now we knew what so many others went through. *Had we ever appreciated our good health? Does anyone?*

Meanwhile, the issue of retirement came up again. Barry's medical practice had become a burden; he didn't feel well enough himself to deal with other people's medical problems. I began to realize that as he felt more ill, it would be up to me to take care of him and also to handle the responsibility of dealing with his practice. The prudent thing seemed to be to retire now, while we both were able to take care of it. I didn't know then that it was already too late for that. We began to make lists of things to do in order to close the practice. I had list upon list, trying to be organized about the many details.

Barry called some of the other local ophthalmologists, to see if anyone would be interested in taking over his practice. Years earlier, younger doctors would have jumped at the chance to take over a thriving practice. But the medical climate had changed. New doctors wanted jobs now; nobody wanted the responsibility of a solo practice. With insurance companies running the show, private practice was much less profitable, and so much more of a hassle that doctors couldn't deal with managing the business of an office as well as the medical side. Still, we had to close the practice. As Barry felt worse and worse, retirement was the right decision for us now.

CHAPTER FIFTY-ONE

DECIDING TO RETIRE

Once we made the decision to retire, I felt relieved, even elated. A burden on my husband's back, and on mine, would soon be gone. Gone; over; finished. No more. No more being tied to the telephone; no more checking in every time we entered or left the house. No more worrying about the thousands of patients' problems. The change was hard to imagine after thirty years of this routine. But there was so much for me to do that I didn't have time to think about all the changes that would occur in my life. At the same time, I was trying to take care of Barry, who still felt sick with his pneumonia. I thought things might be improving, but I wasn't sure.

INTERRUPTION
Nov. - Dec. '01

Barry's health did not improve. We had to figure out what was happening with him. He ended up in our local hospital. So much was going on at once: managing his deteriorating condition, his increasing weakness and the fear of its cause, closing our practice, dealing with our faithful employees, disposing of all the office equipment and furniture, and thirty years of patient records. It was overwhelming.

Most important, however, was Barry's health. And so that was what we dealt with first.

It became a journey, which I could only describe afterwards, looking back from the other side.

****

PART II

LOOKING BACK
TRANSITION

CHAPTER FIFTY-TWO

ALONE
(Jan '02)

It is a Saturday afternoon in January. It is snowing; it is beautiful. This is my first snowfall alone in the house; my house. Not our house any more. Just mine. It is lonely, but it is beautiful nevertheless. I am okay doing the practical things that must get done every day: going shopping, paying the bills, doing the laundry. But just don't show me a sunset, or play music - then I am not okay. I cannot understand how I happen to be here alone like this. What happened? We were waging a terrific battle against this cancer for three and a half years, and yet somehow it won. It took my husband from me, my strong, healthy-looking, stubborn, determined husband; my best friend.

And here I am with my memories of life with Barry. They are wonderful, powerful memories. Well, actually they are both good and bad, happy and not so happy, for we were two normal people who loved each other and had our differences, of course. Still, he was my best friend. Now I face the rest of my life without him. I still feel young, and, if I am lucky, have many years ahead of me. It will soon be time to figure out what I want to do with these years. But right now I am remembering what happened and trying to make it feel real. Trying to get through the days without him. I am doing okay, but it is terribly sad.

My husband took his final journey alone, as we all will. I was privileged to be a witness, as were our children. It was an amazing experience for all of us, but first I will tell you the story of the final weeks.

CHAPTER FIFTY-THREE

RETIREMENT
(Nov '01)

Once we decided to close the practice there was a lot to do. We had to contact all "active" patients, a major undertaking. I sent out the retirement letter Barry had carefully composed months earlier. It began: *"As you may know, I have been fighting a battle with cancer for the past three years. I find that I can no longer devote the energy and attention necessary to practicing ophthalmology. I will, therefore, retire as of December 1, 2001..........I have been very fortunate to have practiced ophthalmology in Northern Westchester for 30 years and to have met and treated so many nice people. I wish you good luck and good health."* Reading the letter made me cry; it was so sad and sincere.

At the same time, we were talking to the other ophthalmologists at the hospital, to see who, if anyone, would be willing to take over the practice. But it seemed that the practice was too large for anyone to assimilate. This was hard to believe, and ironic - we had worked so hard for so many years to build up a large, strong practice, and now nobody wanted it. We knew we had to transfer the patient records and that someone had to assume responsibility for these patients. Finally we came to an agreement with two doctors who were in partnership. Between the two of them, they could absorb our patients into their practice.

Our last day of medical practice is one I will remember forever. It was a Monday morning in November and it was unusually cold outside. The heat in our office building wasn't working that day. Barry wasn't feeling well and the cold office aggravated his discomfort. He could barely stand up straight. He tried valiantly to carry on, but I could see how difficult it was for him. It was too much for him to bear. I was glad we would soon be done with this work.

In the office that morning, it occurred to me that we might not be coming back - ever. At times like this, strange things occur to you, and, although it sounds ludicrous, I suddenly felt that I wanted Barry to give me a Motor Vehicle Form, the paper on which an eye doctor states that your vision is adequate for driving. This form is valid for six months, and I knew I would need it the following spring when I would be renewing my driver's license. Why on earth should such a thing occur to me at a time when I had so many important matters to deal with? I instinctively knew that I did not want to go to any other doctor to have my eyes examined. I think, in addition, that focusing on this trivial matter helped us keep the big picture out of our heads. When I mentioned it to Barry, he agreed immediately, filled out the form and handed it to me. We shared some silent communication about this being the end of our work together in the office. As I held the form he gave me, I had no idea how I would cherish that small piece of paper with his signature; how loathe I would be to finally part with it the following April when I would have to send it to the Department of Motor Vehicles.

While I was taking steps to close our office, I was also coordinating Barry's medical care. His local internist had put him in the hospital after taking one look at him and listening to his chest. He said softly, "I don't like your color," but Barry and I both tried not to hear that comment. This was a sign of things to come: Barry's skin was starting to turn yellow as his liver deteriorated. I thought I had noticed this myself, but was trying to deny it. If Barry's liver was not functioning properly any more, it could only mean one thing: the tumors were taking over the liver.

By now, it was Thanksgiving week-end. We had forgone a big turkey dinner this year. Barry was in the hospital, and Ellen and I were his visitors.

As our patients received Barry's retirement letter, calls and letters started coming in to the office. Every day our secretaries would give us lists of phone calls and piles of cards and letters. They would relay the messages of patients who had stopped in at the office to express their feelings. Everyone was distraught at the thought of losing Barry as their doctor. And they were upset that his deteriorating health was forcing him to close the practice. They truly cared about him.

I hoped Barry felt fortunate in being able to have these letters to read, to know how much his patients valued him. So few people get to hear things like that for it is usually only at a person's funeral that people finally express their appreciation. Too late for the person who really needs to hear it.

CHAPTER FIFTY-FOUR

MEDICAL PROBLEMS

B arry stayed in the hospital for a little over a week. The pneumonia was complicated by asthma, and then by pulmonary emboli. He remained weak, but we thought that once he got home, he would be able to recuperate, and we would still have some time to enjoy our retirement. We knew that people could recover from pneumonia and even from pulmonary emboli.

Barry's weakness did not improve. Still, I reminded myself that he had survived and even thrived through so much. I felt certain that we could deal with pneumonia and pulmonary emboli; we just needed time.

Meanwhile, I was trying to close the office. I couldn't spend time away from Barry, so I was relying on our secretaries to help me more than I wanted to. I had never considered that I would have to close the office without actually being there myself to go through the files, the drawers, the charts, the equipment and instruments. I had thought that Barry and I would work as a team, but that had become impossible.

One day when I had to go out to the bank, I asked a friend to come to the house and sit with Barry. This man had been our friend for over twenty years, and his office was right next door to ours. How difficult it must have been for him to sit in a chair next to Barry's bed, looking at his friend in such weakened condition. I am sure this was something he never expected to have to do. Yet he agreed to help without a moment's hesitation.

It was hard for me to grasp what was happening. With each step down the path, we dealt with a new restriction, a new limitation, without allowing the big picture into our consciousness. Talk about denial: this was the ultimate denial. It was a "we can take it" attitude that had allowed us to do so well through all the past treatments.

Somehow, it was not working any more. There was too much stacked against us, and Barry's body was not strong enough to take it now.

I don't know if he realized what was happening any more than I did. But it didn't matter; we did what we had to do.

I was in denial about the future, yet I was dealing with the tasks at hand. On the last day that I stopped in to check the office, I also visited the local cemetery. I went alone. Barry was no longer able to leave the house. We had discussed the "burial issue" in a general way, and decided that we felt comfortable with the cemetery near our office, a beautiful, small-town graveyard. Its paths were lined with huge old trees, and some of the ancient headstones bore the names of the early settlers in the area. We had enjoyed many long walks there, especially in the summertime when it was shady and cool.

Our discussion of cemetery plots had always been hypothetical. Now the time for action seemed overdue. I met the young cemetery superintendent at the gates, and he showed me plots that were available. The first one he showed me felt right. It was on a little knoll, overlooking the valley where the railroad ran to the city. I knew Barry would like to rest here; he loved the sound of the train whistle. There were trees with birds singing in them. It was beautiful and peaceful. The site was close to the grave of our good friend who had died three years earlier. The cemetery superintendent asked me to come back to his office to sign purchase forms, but I didn't want to be away from Barry for too long. Instead, I leaned against my car as I quickly wrote the check, and hurried home to my ailing husband. I never told Barry what I had done.

In the midst of all this, Dr. Lewis came to our house to visit. *Doctors don't make house calls any more.* This should have tipped us off as to the stage we were in. I'm not sure it did.

It was wonderful to see our doctor, and it was about a month since we had seen him in his office in Manhattan. What a difference this month had made in my husband. Last time, Barry and I had traveled to New York City on the train, and walked from Grand Central Station to the doctor's office. Now it was a major accomplishment for Barry to get out of bed and sit on the couch to meet with the doctor. Dr. Lewis could see what was happening; he told Barry not to bother to get up when he left. He said that he would be back. How that lifted our spirits!

CHAPTER FIFTY-FIVE

THE BEGINNING OF THE END
(Dec '01)

All of a sudden, people were suggesting that we call in Hospice. We didn't know what that entailed. At least I didn't. But when both our local internist and Dr. Lewis made the same suggestion, we followed it. I now realize that these two caring, dedicated men must have been consulting with each other.

Before the hospice workers came, the doctors decided to discontinue Barry's medications. This felt like a drastic measure, an admission of failure. The Thalidomide had contributed to, or even caused, Barry's pulmonary emboli. And yet this drug was our last hope for dealing with the tumors in his liver. Barry had also been on Coumadin for treating the emboli, and it had been impossible to regulate because his liver was not functioning. Therefore, both of these medications had to be discontinued.

I see now that this was the beginning of the end. There was nothing further to try which might stop or even slow down the growth of Barry's tumors.

During his recent hospitalization, Barry had had numerous x-rays, CAT scans, chest scans, and even MRI's, all in an effort to pinpoint the source of his breathing problems. This time neither he nor I had asked to see any of these scans or the reports. We had left that to the doctors. This was in sharp contrast to the way we had religiously reviewed each previous scan. Something told us not to do it now.

I think that if we had looked at the scans during his hospital stay we would have been shocked to see how the tumors were growing. I could see physical evidence of it in Barry's body, but did not bring it to his attention. Of course, there was his yellow skin color. But I had also been alarmed by a bulge on the right side of his back. I hid this observation from Barry. One day, however, I mentioned it to several of the doctors in the hallway outside Barry's hospital room. None of them reacted at all to my statements. I took this to mean that they knew what was happening and there was nothing they could do about it. They were his colleagues and I thought they were having a hard time dealing with it.

By the time Barry came home from this hospital stay and we were preparing for Hospice, I could see that the bulge on the right side of his back was now matched by a similar bulge on the left side. There was only one explanation: the tumors were growing at a fast pace, and were taking up much of his chest. I began to lose hope.

CHAPTER FIFTY-SIX

HOSPICE COMES

The second Wednesday in December 2001, Hospice arrived. A nurse and a social worker came to the house, first met with me, and then visited Barry in the bedroom. They had a lot of information to give me, most of which I was not able to absorb. They did not tell me that I was to be the principal caretaker, the main nurse, the decision-maker, the guide for my husband on his final journey. So much was coming at me all at once, that I didn't have a moment to recognize the huge change that had occurred. We were no longer looking for improvement, or even stabilization; we were just hoping to keep Barry comfortable.

The hospice workers produced a paper for me to sign: the "DNR." This was the "Do Not Resuscitate" form. At that moment, I was horrified at the thought. This paper instructed any emergency health worker to let Barry die, not to resuscitate him. I balked at signing: I still wanted to try to save him. A few minutes later, in the bedroom, when the nurse and social worker introduced themselves to Barry, his first question was, "Where's the DNR?" When he willingly signed it, the nurse whispered to the social worker, "I knew she didn't understand."

With each small step, a little more reality crept into my consciousness. But I was so preoccupied with the details of meeting Barry's daily needs that I didn't see the enormity of the change. Did he? One afternoon, he said, "I didn't even get one day of retirement." I had no answer.

As Barry weakened physically, he mellowed. I could see him letting go of the controlling attitude he had assumed ever since I had known him. I knew that he felt responsible for me and for our daughters, but now that he couldn't bear that responsibility any longer, he softened. He gave it up and became accepting.

It was December; the holidays were coming. Sara and Richard were scheduled to arrive from Alaska in about a week. I wondered if Barry would still be in shape to talk to them by then. I was keeping my fingers crossed.

The hospice nurse came to the house twice a week. She tried her best to show me how to use the oxygen machine, the back-up oxygen tanks, the nebulizer, and myriad new medications designed to keep Barry comfortable. Some of this I picked up right away. Some I scoffed at, not believing that we would actually need such contraptions. The first time they tried to deliver the hospital bed, Barry refused it, saying that he didn't need it. Little did we know that when they returned with it within a few days, we would be desperate for it.

In the midst of all this, Dr. Lewis arrived for another visit. This time, Barry had to stay in bed to receive him; there was no question of his even sitting up. The doctor was his usual cheerful self, offering to help in any way, to be available for us at any time. This must have been awful for him, a man who had become our friend, who respected Barry and who had guided us both through the past three and a half years. Whatever his personal feelings, Dr. Lewis showed us only a smile and compassion.

About this same time, our local internist also came to visit. I was astounded. Although he and Barry were colleagues and friends, he had never been to our house. All this interest gave Barry and me great comfort. By this time, I was not leaving Barry alone at all, which meant that I was not leaving the house. Period. I had to call on friends to do chores for me, and Ellen was helping out in any way she could. I was so grateful for all of this, but it was a new and challenging role for me, one of asking people for help.

I recall one particularly stressful day for me. Barry and I were alone in the house and he was unable to get out of bed any more. There was a storm raging outside: wind and rain pounded the house. We were using the oxygen from time to time. I was still not very familiar with the machine, but I managed. Since we live in a quiet area outside of town we frequently lose electrical power during storms. On that day, I became terrified that we would lose power, the oxygen machine would not work, and I would have to drag the back-up oxygen tanks upstairs and try to figure out how to use them, all in the dark. I felt desperately alone, and solely responsible for our welfare.

CHAPTER FIFTY-SEVEN

THE LAST WEEKS

Every day now seemed to bring a great change in my husband. Although his physical condition diminished, his mental clarity did not. Barry remained alert, and he became peaceful and accepting. We had entered an unknown place. I felt that we were players on a stage; the script was written for us to enact; we each had our role. We did our best. Somehow, we knew we had to.

Then it was Chanukah: the Festival of Lights. Ellen came up from the city with gifts for her father. He smiled as she opened them for him. One package held a beautiful, warm, navy-blue fleece pullover. Barry loved it, but he said to me quietly, "When am I ever going to wear this?" I told him he didn't have to wear it - it was good enough to just feel it and enjoy it.

The night we moved Barry into a hospital bed, our younger daughter Sara and her husband were scheduled to arrive from Alaska. We had been promised that the bed would be delivered all day; but it never came. By evening I was frantic, calling both the hospice office and the hospital bed delivery company. Barry was uncomfortable propped up on pillows in a regular bed any more. He needed a bed that could be adjusted; he couldn't support himself. It was ten o'clock at night when the bed finally arrived. It had to be assembled, and, more difficult, someone had to transfer Barry into it, since he could no longer walk, nor support himself standing up. Between the night-call hospice nurse, and a friend who was a nurse herself, we managed the task. At last, Barry was settled into a bed where he could be comfortable, where his head and feet could be adjusted without any effort on his part.

Once he was in the hospital bed, it became essential to Barry to be able to see the view outside the sliding glass doors in our bedroom. This was the way our bed had always faced, and we had both enjoyed looking out at the woods behind our house while we rested in bed. Now it was more important than ever for Barry to have this view; he wanted to make every minute count. We pushed the bedroom furniture around until there was room for the hospital bed next to our regular bed; now he could lie there and enjoy the scenery. As he did, he said to me softly, in wonderment, "I'll never leave this room."

There was excitement as our Alaska family arrived, and I was grateful that Barry was still alert. It was wonderful to see Sara and Richard. Although it was late at night, we all were so happy to see each other that nobody wanted to go to sleep. My prayers had been answered: Barry had been able to talk with both of his daughters and his son-in-law.

By this time, my brother Bruce and his family arrived for their holiday visit with us, and I really needed their help. I planned to use them to go to our office and to complete the chores involved in closing the practice. I had been instructing our secretaries, who brought bags of folders, papers, and supplies to me at the house daily, but I had not set foot in the office myself in weeks. When people came to the office to look at the equipment we needed to get rid of, I had to handle the arrangements over the telephone. The situation at home made the job of closing the office unbelievably difficult. Everyone was being flexible and helpful, and I cannot express how much I appreciated it.

In addition to all this, we were all worried about my mother: should we bring her over to say good-bye to Barry, or would she find it too distressing? It wasn't right to leave her out of this experience, but we didn't want to cause her any harm. Finally, we worked out a plan where my brother would bring her to the house, and she would have time to visit with Barry and the rest of the family, including her granddaughter from Alaska. It worked out well, and my mother was able to contain her grief and to say good-bye. I tried to put myself in Mom's shoes, and wondered how I would deal with the terminal illness of a member of the younger generation, but I found it too awful to contemplate.

CHAPTER FIFTY-EIGHT

FINAL DAYS: THE SPIRITUAL JOURNEY

In his last days, Barry was unable to eat without assistance. It surprised me that he still cared about food, but he surely did. He wanted vanilla ice-cream every day, and he asked for other favorites, especially scrambled eggs and "smoothies" that I made with fruit and ice-cream. One of my mother's friends made a cheesecake and sent it over with her. Cheesecake seemed too heavy to give to Barry. I thought it would give him indigestion. But when he heard "cheesecake," his eyes lit up. He was the same old Barry. When his eyes widened and he said, "Cheesecake," I told him gently that cheesecake wouldn't be good for him now. But he turned to me with a look that said, "I want that cheesecake!" I fed Barry cheesecake that day and he loved every bite of it. It makes me smile, even now.

Hospice sent a nurse's aide to help for twelve hours during the day, but I was uncomfortable leaving Barry with her. His skin had become extremely sensitive and I didn't feel that she was gentle enough with him. Though I turned to her for her knowledge about patients in this stage of life, I continued to give Barry his medications and to bathe him, and I insisted that the aide not handle him in any way without my supervision. This did not make it easy between us. But the most important thing was my role of making sure Barry was as comfortable as possible.

Barry was doing something in his mind in these last few days. He seemed to be occupied elsewhere, and had become extremely peaceful. He had been a classic, hard-driving, "Type-A" person his whole life. Now he became accepting, non-judgmental, and philosophical. Several of us saw him smiling at times, with his eyes closed, as he seemed to be remembering or working things out in his mind. It was as if he was someplace else, and then he would come back to us.

He spoke individually to various family members, softly dispensing wise thoughts to them: advice about living a balanced life. He told our college-aged nephew to be sure he didn't let work become his whole life. He told my cousin to be sure she lived life every day, not saving enjoyment for those few weeks of vacation she took. Barry had always been smart; but now he was wise as well. Something big was going on, and we were deeply impressed with the sanctity of this experience. We felt as if we were Barry's stewards, here to help him with his transition. We took it as our job to ease his way, to provide for his last earthly needs while he was still tied to his physical body. It was a humbling experience, one that is hard to describe. I had never seen anything like this in my life, and it changed me. Something was going on that I didn't understand. I felt, along with my family, that we were privileged to witness this transition, that Barry was giving all of us a parting gift.

During the final days, Barry stopped eating and drinking, and although I found this distressing, Dr. Lewis encouraged me to let Barry do whatever he wanted. This was comforting. My instincts told me this, but it was reassuring to hear it from a trusted authority. By now, our doctor was calling us every day, sometimes more than once, to keep up with Barry's condition and to give us any guidance we needed. I am sure he knew exactly what was going on, and what stage we were in. Even though I was at my husband's side every day, I was so numb that the finality of it didn't register.

We played Barry's favorite music softly for him: recordings of the young guitar player we had met in Sedona. Barry recognized the music, smiled and enjoyed it.

I had never seen anything so moving, so peaceful, in all my life. I don't know what I expected, but certainly not this. Barry was leaving; he was saying good-bye to his life on earth, and the people he loved. He had stopped being concerned with his body, with earthly matters, and had turned his attention inward, to some process going on in his mind.

Inexplicable things were occurring at home at the same time. One night, I awakened in the middle of the night trembling all over.

I felt cold, and my entire body was shaking. I got up and raised the heat, put some warmer clothing on, and went back to sleep. The clock read "12:00." The next morning at breakfast, my daughter said that she had awakened in the middle of the night feeling sick. It had been around midnight, she said, and she had felt strangely ill, but had fallen asleep again. I told her about my experience at exactly the same time. This sort of thing happened several more times during Barry's last few days. Ellen and I felt the same sort of physical discomfort at the same times. One day we were not even in the same town when it happened. This is one of the things that I have no explanation for, but I feel that it was no coincidence. Perhaps Barry had been having some physical distress at those times, perhaps breathing trouble, and somehow we were connected. This sounds impossible, yet it occurred to us both.

All this time, I had my family helping me, staying at the house, comforting me. My two daughters and my son-in-law were my constant companions, as were my brother and his wife and children. I felt their support and I leaned on them. They made this difficult time bearable for me. They helped me with everything from shopping and cooking to holding Barry's hand and sharing my tears. One day, Bruce and Jane decided that I needed some fresh air; I hadn't been out of the house in many days. They convinced me to take a walk with them on our road. I agreed reluctantly and I gingerly made my way down the street, with both of them by my side. After going a short distance, I became so anxious that I had to turn around and go back. I was afraid to be away from Barry at this critical time. My brother and his wife understood. I don't know what I would have done without them. And I know they wanted to be part of this experience with Barry and with me.

CHAPTER FIFTY-NINE

THE END
(Dec. 28 '01)

Sara and Richard had to end their visit and return to Alaska. They were reluctant to leave, but we didn't know how long Barry would linger, and they couldn't stay indefinitely. They left with heavy hearts, but happy to have witnessed such a peaceful experience, and to have had the chance to say good-bye to their father. Our older daughter, Ellen, told me that she didn't think Barry would "leave" as long as his two daughters were at home. She also had been away from her job for some time, so I convinced her to go back to the city for a day, go to work, and return the following day. She agreed, saying that she felt at peace now. She believed that her leaving the house would allow her father to pass on.

My husband's last day with us was a Thursday, the day after the children had gone home. When I gave Barry some medication at 4 A.M., I asked him to open his mouth, and he did, although his eyes were closed. That was the last time Barry responded to me. He was sleeping peacefully from then on, quite deeply, perhaps in a semi-comatose state. When it was time for the next dose of medicine at 8 A.M., he didn't respond when I asked him to open his mouth. By then his breathing was irregular, and his pulse was weak and hard to find. But we weren't bothering with that sort of thing any more. Our doctor had said it wasn't important, and we understood him.

Our hope that day was to keep Barry comfortable, peaceful, to whisper words of love and peace to him, hoping he could hear us. I told him from my heart that he had done a good job; his work here was done; he could let go now.

On that last day, as much as I wanted contact with Barry, I didn't want to touch his skin at all. He was peaceful, lying there comfortably, his mind occupied elsewhere. I felt that if I touched him, I would bring him back. He would be reminded of his body, of this earth, of the place he was leaving. It didn't seem right to interrupt his inner journey.

Dr. Lewis called that morning, and when I said that Barry wasn't responsive, he said that he would try to stop by that afternoon. Late that afternoon the doorbell rang: it was our guardian angel. We ushered him into the bedroom, where everything was hushed, holy, and peaceful. He stood at the bedside, taking everything in at a glance. Here was the man who had guided us through almost four years of surgery, radiation, chemotherapy, and procedures, good responses to treatment and bad ones, the man we had spoken to every week no matter where in the world his work had taken him. How did he feel, looking down at his patient, his friend, who now was so far away from us all?

Dr. Lewis knew exactly what we all needed. He did not speak to Barry at all. This was shocking to me. During every other visit, Dr. Lewis had focused primarily on his patient; now he didn't speak a word to him. I am sure that if he had thought that his voice could have brought Barry any comfort at all, he would have addressed him. But Dr. Lewis knew more than we did. He spoke to me, and to my brother, who was helping me, as we stood at the bed. He told us that this was the way it was supposed to be. He reassured us that we were doing the right things; and he said he would call us soon. I felt certain that he wanted me to call him if anything changed.

Before we went to sleep that night, I dismissed the hospice aide. There was nothing more she could do for us. Barry's breathing and the oxygen machine were making a lot of noise. Dr. Lewis had said, "You aren't sleeping in here with this noise, are you?" So that night, I went to sleep across the hall from Barry. But all the bedroom doors were left wide open; we were all on alert.

I awoke with a start in the middle of the night. The clock said, "12:54." Chills went down my spine; "1254" was the phone number of the Emergency Room at our local hospital. I had dialed that number every time Barry had been called by the Emergency Room for the past thirty years. A red "1254" blinked at me in the dark. And it was very quiet in the house. Perhaps the quiet was what had awakened me. I could hear the oxygen machine, but I couldn't hear my husband breathing. I got up and walked across the hall into our bedroom. The night light shone. And I could clearly see that Barry's chest was not rising and falling. He was not breathing. He was not breathing.

CHAPTER SIXTY

AFTER THE END

He was not breathing. He must be dead. I had never been alone with a dead person before. This was my husband, my best friend for forty years. But it was also clear that this was not Barry at all. My husband had been here a few hours before, but he was not here now. There was an empty body on the bed, and my husband was gone. What lay on the bed was some physical body that my husband had inhabited, had worn like a suit of clothes; but that physical entity lying on the bed, motionless, was certainly not my husband.

His head was turned slightly to the left, and his mouth was slightly open, as if the breath of life had just escaped. I called my brother, and he and his wife got up and came into the room. Barry still had the oxygen tube on; I went to him and removed it from his nose. His forehead was cold. The tube for the oxygen was looped around his arm, and I when I picked up his hand, it was still warm. His feet were warm, too. He must have just died.

I couldn't stop looking at the body. The body lying on the bed, the body which had been my husband so recently. What had happened that made such a profound difference in this living being? So many things work in conjunction to keep us alive. When the balance tips, and the forces working against life get too strong, what happens?

My mind went to the practical matters at hand. My brother, being a doctor, got out a stethoscope. I got a mirror to hold up in front of my husband's mouth. My brother also felt for a pulse. As if we needed any of that. It was all too clear.

It felt essential to have my family with me. What if this had happened at any time other than this holiday time, when we always visited with each other? So many things were happening to make this easier for me; difficult as it was, it could have been so much worse, I know.

CHAPTER SIXTY-ONE

THE NEXT FEW DAYS

When we were very sure that Barry was gone, we called Hospice. By then it was the middle of the night, but the hospice nurse on call had to come to pronounce my husband dead. She also had to remove all the remaining narcotic medications. She was followed by the men from the funeral parlor, who took Barry's body away. Suddenly this seemed so final. When I said something to that effect, the men asked me if I wanted a few minutes with him. That made no sense to me. I had just had a lifetime with Barry. This empty body on the bed was not my husband. Nevertheless, once the body had been taken away, there was nothing left of my husband at all.

I was exhausted; I sat down at the kitchen table in wonderment. It is hard to grasp reality at a time like that. I found myself strangely hungry, and craved chocolate ice-cream. Bruce and Jane and their son were with me, and they understood comfort food. Within a few minutes, we were all sitting around the kitchen table eating ice-cream. Barry would have loved that. On our very first date, almost forty-one years before, on our day off from camp, we had gotten a container of ice-cream and two spoons and gone to a state park to picnic. This was truly the right thing to do now.

By then it was 3:30 A.M., and we all knew we would have to try to get some sleep because the next day would bring lots of things to take care of. Before I went to bed, I called Sara and Richard. Alaska is four hours behind us in time, so it was 11:30 P.M. there, and I knew they would want to make plans to come back east for the funeral. Even as I spoke to my daughter, I could hardly believe what I was saying. The one thing we had been dreading for almost four years had happened.

Early the next morning, I started making phone calls. I didn't want to tell my mother while she was alone, so I called my cousin who lived near her and asked if she or her husband could go to my mother's house and tell her. Then I called Ellen in New York City; she would take an early train back to us. The next person I called was our Dr. Lewis. He had been waiting for my call. In fact, he said he had been trying to reach me, but the phone line had been busy. It was wonderful to hear his comforting voice.

The next days were a blur of calling friends and relatives, making decisions at the funeral home, and preparing for the funeral and burial. It all seemed unreal; how could this be happening? How could I be doing all this without my partner? I felt too young to be in this position, yet I was not alone. Everywhere I turned, people were being kind and supportive to me.

CHAPTER SIXTY-TWO

FUNERAL

The day of the funeral arrived, and I had my family with me: my two daughters, my son-in-law, my brother and his family, and my mother. My cousin and her family had brought my mother over, and were being sure to stay near her, so I knew she was taken care of. I was in a daze, unable to believe what was happening.

So many people showed up at the funeral parlor: all sorts of friends, swimming friends of ours, karate friends of mine, my husband's colleagues from the hospital, nurses as well as doctors, our relatives, some of whom had flown in from distant places, our first chemo nurse, our second chemo nurse, my karate Sensei, even patients who somehow had found out. Later, people told me that the line to get into the funeral home had stretched around the block. Barry would have been dumbfounded. One of our chemo nurses was working at the hospital, two blocks away, that Sunday. She had gotten someone from the Emergency Room to relieve her, and had hurried down to the funeral home, making her way through the line to get inside. The thought of this soft-spoken, diminutive woman pushing her way through the crowd was both astonishing and touching.

Later at the nearby cemetery, I watched as a long line of people waited to throw a shovelful of dirt down onto the casket, after it had been lowered into the grave. This ancient ritual seemed so meaningful to me. These people were helping to bury a friend.

Many, many people came back to the house to pay their respects; they stayed for hours. We sat together, talking about the unreality of it all, remembering good times, and trying to comfort each other. It was somber, but still a party in honor of my husband, and everyone there had fond memories. I felt that they all wanted to help me get through this time of sorrow.

When everyone had left, I was alone with my two daughters and my son-in-law. Soon it would be New Year's Eve, a time of new beginnings, and a time of a new role for me. I was alone at the head of my little family, alone in the house, without my partner, but still feeling him very much with me.

Ellen, Sara, and Richard had a few days to spend with me before they had to return to their lives and their responsibilities. We had time for a trip to the Connecticut beach on Long Island Sound that Barry and I always enjoyed so much. It was a cold, windy day, but an emotional and beautiful experience. I was with the people I loved most in the world. We were all shaken from the events of the past couple of weeks, but happy to be alive and together, and to be visiting a place Barry had loved.

And then, before I knew it, I was really alone. My family left, and I was alone in our house - my house. I knew I had to have some sort of structure in my life, but because I had no job now, I had to make my own schedule. My life; my new life. My old life had had so much routine in it, and now I had none. I was feeling my way in the dark. Swimming and karate provided some semblance of structure, and I was grateful that at least I had that.

There were many details to deal with concerning the estate, closing the practice, and other financial matters. I needed social contact now that I was away from a job. I started making arrangements to meet with other single women I knew, who were either widowed or divorced. There seemed to be a lot of people in a similar position to mine, and it was good for me to see them coping and dealing with life, and even enjoying many activities. There is a tendency to feel that one shouldn't enjoy life too much after a loss. The first morning I caught myself humming, I was taken aback and yet I felt it was a milestone. I saw the road to recovery.

One evening a swimming friend of ours, Sister Elaine, organized a memorial ceremony for Barry at the Boys' Club, where we had been exercising for years. The "early morning swimmers," as we called ourselves, gathered together, and Sister Elaine provided candles, music, and snacks, and we remembered Barry. Each person recalled a specific memory of him to relate to the group; a few of these stories were quite funny. Some of them were about heated discussions that had taken place in the men's locker room, which Barry had described to me, but which none of the other women there knew about. There was one man there who had regularly engaged Barry in a political argument. My husband had taken these arguments lightly, but his friend had been serious about them and regularly got quite worked up; it was amusing. One of the women at the ceremony hadn't really known Barry, but remembered seeing him waiting for me outside after our swim every day, waiting and waiting. We laughed a lot, and also cried. Barry had been such an integral member of our group.

I must not forget the essential support I received from Dr. Lewis. He called me frequently at first, offering sympathy and encouragement. I realized later how hard this must have been for him; after all, he had lost someone who meant a lot to him. I guess he could tell that I was doing okay, because after a while, his calls became less frequent. He told me later that he had avoided calling because I had needed some time to myself to work things out. He gave me the space and a little push to stand up on my own. It is tempting to lean on someone when you are hurting, but you really have to make your own way in the world. It definitely can be done, but it cannot be done without pain. One day, Dr. Lewis said that it would be hard, but it is meant to be. *Of course! It is meant to be. If it wasn't hard, then the loss would have meant nothing.*

CHAPTER SIXTY-THREE

A NEW ROLE
(Early 2002)

The days passed. I muddled through. I had swimming and karate. Exercise helped, but I was too distracted to work on any art in my studio. I was in survival mode. I met friends for lunch, walks, movies, dinner, anything. I was afraid not to. I was running to keep from thinking. I was afraid to be alone.

For a while I avoided places I'd shared with Barry, but you can't do that forever. Gradually I returned to the local diner, the shops. I took a walk where we had strolled, but I felt as if people were staring at me and how alone I was. It was hard to meet friends or patients who didn't know that Barry had died. It was hard to say the words. And I spent time with other widows, women who had lived through it, who were still alive and were enjoying life, who could advise me or answer questions I had.

I had two big questions on my mind: where to live and whether to get a job. I knew that I couldn't make rational decisions yet. And Dr. Lewis urged me to take my time. Somehow, his calm advice gave me permission to slow down and not to rush into anything. Although I was hurting inside and lonely, I knew that things could be worse, and I didn't want to jump into anything.

As I fell into a routine, I began to relax and feel more comfortable. It wasn't a shock to realize that I was alone, living alone, cooking for one, taking care of things by myself. This is not to say that I didn't cry a lot, but I knew I needed to let out the sadness. The feeling of panic that had been my constant companion, took a vacation now and then. I saw other people who were living alone by choice, and that was reassuring.

I wondered if I would ever return to the places Barry and I had loved to visit: the Grand Canyon, Rockport, Ithaca. I loved visiting these places and I wanted to go back, but when and how? I trusted that I would find the answers to these questions with time. I still felt tremendous support and love from my family and close friends, and, of course, from Dr. Lewis. I knew I was lucky.

Then there was the sense of my husband's presence. I felt him with me. I found that other widows understood this feeling. Before Barry's death, I hadn't believed in God, in what the Bible says, or in any sort of afterlife. Now I wondered. I felt that there was much more to human beings than we knew, more than we could possibly understand. Barry seemed to have learned so much in his final days. He had become peaceful and accepting. I believed that he was at peace now, that somehow he was okay, and that he had not slipped into nothingness, which is what I would have said six months earlier. I cannot explain how I came to change my view, except to say that I had been a witness to Barry's final journey, and had been awed and humbled by what I saw. Barry had been preparing for a transition. It was clear that this was something very important, and it was a miracle that my husband was moving through it in such a peaceful manner. I realized, after talking to others who had suffered losses, how lucky Barry and I and our family had been.

Slowly, I felt myself begin to look toward my future. I still felt my loss terribly, but knew that I did have a future on this earth. I was here, still alive. I began to want more than just to get through the days, although living through this raw time was necessary for healing. I gave myself permission to take my time to deal with my loss and to do whatever seemed right for me. I also realized that the right things to do would become evident if I just relaxed and let them unfold. I began to have faith in my ability to cope.

CHAPTER SIXTY-FOUR

SPRING 2002

How can you explain how it feels to miss someone? Someone you have been with for forty years, someone who has been your best friend, the person you shared just about everything with? Someone you met when you were eighteen, someone you grew with, loved and argued with, someone you expected to grow old with? Someone who was truly your partner? Someone who started out with you defying the college dormitory rules, coming in late, being "daring," and who eventually married you and became the stable provider, the rule-maker for your children, epitomizing the very things you both had rebelled against? And someone who was your final ally in the biggest fight of your lives, the three-and-a-half-year battle to the death with cancer?

Words fail. You get up and go through the days, but there is a black hole inside. You do meaningful things, enjoy a blue sky or a sunset, but all the while there is this hole. Then you begin to love the hole and you don't want to get over it, even as it diminishes. All the while, you have to survive. You have no control over all this. It just happens.

With the promise of spring, I felt happy to be alive. I didn't feel alone. I was grateful for the beautiful ending Barry had experienced and shared with us. I felt part of a spiritual whole.

Many practical matters were looming and had to be addressed. I spent the next few months trying to formulate plans. I didn't know whether to move into the middle of town or to stay in my house on a quiet road. Should I stay alone way out there? Barry and I had thought I would not, but I needed to find a place I felt comfortable in, one with the beauty of nature that surrounded my house. The thought of moving was daunting. Then, I wondered: should I get a job? Maybe volunteer? I also needed to find a financial advisor and to get my accounts in order. All of this would take time and a clear head.

Meanwhile, in March, Sara and Richard came to visit from Alaska, relieving me from all these concerns. I spent a week with them and with Ellen. We had shared an extraordinary spiritual experience and we felt a deep bond. One day, while the four of us were sitting in Grand Central Station, I had a revelation. I had been thinking about a headstone for Barry's grave, and had been wracking my brain for just the right inscription. As I sat there surrounded by the people I loved most in the world, the answer suddenly came to me. I would put the image of Red Rock Crossing at the top of the stone! Red Rock Crossing, a spot in the red mountains in Sedona, Arizona, was our favorite place in our favorite town in our favorite part of the country. Barry's body would rest forever beneath the red rocks, the place where we had expected to retire.

I also found the perfect reading for the unveiling ceremony, a ritual we would hold at the one-year mark, when the headstone was set. I had been searching for an appropriate piece to read, and my daughter Ellen came up with just the thing. She said something told her to look at John Steinbeck's work. So I started going through Steinbeck's books, and found that at the end of *Cannery Row*, the protagonist, a doctor, reviews his life as he stands at his sink washing dishes. How perfect. As soon as Barry became ill, he took over the task of washing dishes in our house. He said he wanted to be useful and to help me since I was doing a lot more work now, taking care of him. Steinbeck's piece was just the thing, especially since he was Barry's favorite author. Things were falling into place.

Dr. Lewis visited me a few times early on. He gave me moral support, and believed that I had the strength to go on. His faith in me gave me courage. I also had the pleasure of giving him something Barry had worn and loved that I wanted him to have: it was a Native American watchband Dr. Lewis had noticed on Barry's wrist on one of our first visits to Sloan-Kettering. Dr. Lewis had been fascinated with its unusual design and had asked Barry about it. It makes me happy to know that something Barry used every day now belongs to the man who gave us hope and guidance for so long.

CHAPTER SIXTY-FIVE

MY BIRTHDAY
(April 2002)

Forever stretched out in front of me, long and lonely. There were good days and bad days. I spent my fifth-ninth birthday in Virginia with Bruce and Jane, two of the people who helped me through Barry's final days. We spent a long weekend of hiking, kayaking, talking for hours, remembering Barry. It was a good way for me to celebrate my birthday. This was the first birthday I had not spent with Barry since I had been eighteen. I had had forty birthdays with him.

As my new life began to take on some semblance of regularity, I began to get used to being alone. I started a volunteer job at a cancer center in the local hospital. This was difficult, but something told me to do it. I was learning to listen to my instincts. I spent my time at the hospital talking to the cancer patients in their rooms, getting them items they needed from the kitchen, or just sitting with them. There were a surprising number of patients who didn't seem to have any visitors. I felt that I was making a difference, and knew how grateful Barry would have felt if someone had stopped in to talk to him when he was alone in his hospital room.

I also started reading books about grief, about widows, survival, life after cancer, and how people coped with loss. It was comforting that I was not the only one in this position. I still did not like living alone, but could not even conceive of sharing my life with someone new. So I resigned myself to being single and enjoying everything I could, to remembering all the good things I had had in my life, and trying not to waste the time I had left.

****

PART III

LIVING ON

Chapter Sixty-Six

Memorial Week-End
(2002)

Memorial Day week-end, 2002 was exactly four years after Barry and I had visited Sara and Richard in Seattle. Four years after we had first noticed the lump in Barry's leg. Everything had changed at that moment. Four years is a long time, and yet how I wish it had been much longer.

Memorial Day week-end 2002: five months after Barry's death, five long months that I had been living on my own. I felt raw and panicky at times, but not all the time. Part of me wanted to get on with things, and another part wanted to never get over what happened. Never. I refused to accept it, but still had stopped listening for Barry's step on the stairs. This was a strange kind of limbo: can't go back, and don't want to go forward.

During the early grieving process, feelings of anger and resentment rose up in me. I felt angry at Barry for conflicts we had never resolved. But I wasn't angry at him for dying, as the books on grieving predicted. How could I resent him for leaving when I knew how much he wanted to stay and how hard he fought to live? In the past we had our differences over issues like raising our children and relating to various family members. We had each been convinced that we were right. This led to resentment in me, and I am sure Barry felt the same way. Now I was left to deal with this anger and somehow integrate it with my grief.

I tried various techniques recommended by friends and grief counselors. I wrote letters to Barry. I yelled at him when I was driving alone in the car. I even had conversations with him as I fell asleep. Two evenings as I spoke to him while sitting up in bed, the bathroom light started blinking at me. If this was Barry answering me, I didn't get it. I worked hard to achieve forgiveness, but it eluded me. Finally, I turned my attention to other things, and focused on making a new life.

My volunteer work at the local cancer center was rewarding, but challenging. It was hard to see the cancer patients, but the setting was so familiar. And I saw that my work there made a difference to the patients lying in those beds. I could provide some small comfort to them. Perhaps this work was something that would help me through this transition period. Perhaps it was where my future lay. I didn't know yet.

I began making plans for my summer. Certain adventures seemed to drop into my lap, and I took a chance and said YES.

The first was a trip to my nephew's college graduation in Cambridge. Bruce and Jane invited me to join them to celebrate their son's accomplishment. The second offer came from Barry's cousin, who asked if I would like to join her at Cornell's summer program in July. After a brief hesitation, I eagerly agreed. My last trip would be to Montana, where I would meet Sara and Richard to give them Barry's car to take back with them to Alaska. Three adventures; the beginning of stepping back into the world. On my own, but with family for support.

I was excited about these plans, and believed I would be taking Barry's spirit with me. I felt sure that I was not alone. That was something that I did not expect. But then again, I don't know what I did expect.

How could I know for four years that my husband had a terrible disease, that the statistics were bad, and still not think about the ultimate outcome? How could I expect to beat the odds, even when treatment after treatment proved futile? So many times Barry said to me, that first summer, even before we knew his diagnosis, "If this is sarcoma, then I'm a dead man." I thought he was just being pessimistic, or expressing his worst fears. I never believed he would turn out to be right. I couldn't conceive of life without him.

I was not the only one who felt this way about Barry. Several friends and even some of his patients told me that they couldn't believe he was gone. He was such a presence, such a strong person, such a large personality. He loved to talk, to laugh, to engage people, to experience life. He never left well enough alone; he was always trying to shake things up. It is hard to understand how someone like that could simply be gone from this earth. You knew Barry had been here. He left some big footprints behind.

CHAPTER SIXTY-SEVEN

THREE SUMMER JOURNEYS

Summer 2002 was wonderful for me, despite my fears and bouts of loneliness. I ventured out, tried new things, traveled with new companions. I felt daring; I felt excited.

In early June, Bruce and Jane took me with them to Cambridge for their son's college graduation. I was able to travel with them, away from my house and all my familiar, comforting things. Traveling with family was the only way I could have ventured out just then. At the graduation, I marveled at all the talented young adults about to embark on their life-voyages. What a magical time of life that is.

During the commencement ceremony, the heavens opened and rain poured down on the graduates, their parents and friends. We all sat outside in puddles on our chairs, and little waterfalls poured down on our heads from our neighbors' umbrellas. I thought it was great fun, but a little voice in the back of my head reminded me that Barry would not have liked it as much.

My brother and his wife and I stayed in a hotel near the Harvard campus. This was the first time I had stayed in a hotel room by myself without Barry. I felt vulnerable and scared and terribly alone. Yet I was glad to have been included in this celebration. It was a good first trip for me, an experiment, testing the waters of travel without Barry but with family. Who would ever imagine that your baby brother and his wife would be the ones to help you emerge from the despair of widowhood? I could remember when Barry and I drove my brother and his then-girlfriend, Jane, to school dances when they were high school sweethearts. Now they were leading me back into the world.

I wanted to take a side trip to Rockport, an hour away on Cape Ann. I hoped to revisit the town Barry and I had loved, and had spent so many happy days in. Bruce, Jane, and their son asked to come with me, so we spent an afternoon there together. I took time to walk the paths that were so familiar, to stroll by the wharf and docks. It was drizzling and cool: the weather I like best. Jane and I amused ourselves by shopping for gifts, and laughed a lot at how much we were buying. We browsed in Barry's favorite pewter shop. It was a great distraction from all the memories.

A month later, I started out on my next adventure, a week at Cornell University. When Barry's cousin first asked if I would attend a summer program on finance and investing with her, I was taken aback. But after thinking it over, I decided to do it. This week was just what I needed: a new experience in an old familiar setting. This was the place Barry and I had chosen to spend our final week-end away before he became too sick to travel. I was lucky to be spending time with someone who had known Barry her whole life, and could appreciate how I was feeling.

I was nervous as I made the four-hour-drive to Ithaca alone, wending my way along country roads through upstate New York. This was the longest drive I had made by myself since Barry's death. I kept feeling that if something happened to me, nobody would ever know.

I stopped halfway to eat at the Roscoe Diner, where Barry and I had stopped every time we had driven to Ithaca. I sat at the counter, ordered a snack, and was served by the same elderly waitress who had brought us food so many times. I fought back tears as memories flooded my mind.

Back on the road, I tried to relax. I drove through beautiful countryside, past lovely old farms, ramshackle houses, and little villages. Some of the farmhouses were in disrepair, since upstate New York was having hard times. It had been this way for years. I had traveled these roads in every season, but never alone.

When the road entered Ithaca, I began to get excited. It was the same feeling I had experienced so often; I had been coming to this town for more than fifty years. When I was a child, my family had driven here every summer on the way to my father's relatives in Niagara Falls. Later, when I attended college here, I had been thrilled to live in a place with such natural beauty. It was the first time I had ever lived away from home, and it was the perfect place to grow and learn.

Now I found myself at Cornell again and on my own. I unloaded my gear and found the way to my assigned room in one of the new dormitories. Then I went downstairs to wait for Barry's cousin to arrive. What an assortment of people were here for the various week-long seminars. I felt self-conscious. It was as if I had a big sign on my back that read "I am alone." But I forced myself to smile and to act "normal." This was the beginning of a new me stepping out into the world.

During the week at Cornell, I got up very early in the morning when the air still had its nighttime chill, and walked the campus by myself, before everyone else was awake. The only other people I saw were the members of a sports team, on their early-morning workout. I enjoyed the special beauty of this private time on the campus. I needed to be alone, to remember, and to work things out in my mind.

On two of the mornings, a great blue heron accompanied me, and then swooped down into the gorge as I watched him from a high bridge. It was breathtaking, and I could enjoy it in solitude, feeling my husband's spirit with me. I sat on the stone bench overlooking Cayuga Lake, where Barry and I had spent hours daydreaming. I stood on the spot where he had asked me to marry him, thirty-eight years earlier. I could linger as long as I liked. I was in no rush. I closed my eyes and smelled the summer air, listening to the birds and the wind. By the time I got back to the dormitory, the other summer school participants were getting up and when I joined them for breakfast, I was feeling renewed and ready for our classes.

I visited Risley Hall, my old freshman dormitory, and the classroom buildings I had spent so much time in years ago, before I had even met Barry. I climbed the familiar stairs, with their deep grooves worn down by generations of students. I strolled along the age-old paths across the quad under the huge trees. I could remember doing this by myself, and then later with Barry so many times.

The class I was taking was held in Sage Hall, a renovated building that had once been a women's dormitory. Sage Hall was the very dorm in which my mother had lived when she was a student here. This triggered many emotions in me, and signaled both a return to my roots and a new beginning.

The week at Cornell was filled with new experiences. I slept in a single room in a new dorm, and I could hear the comforting voices of students outside in the summer night as I was falling asleep. The summer program participants had meals in a large modern dining hall, cafeteria-style, with all sorts of good food - quite a contrast from the formal dining of my college days. Now we sat at large round tables, meeting different people at each meal. There was time for all sorts of informal discussion. Afternoons were free, as were evenings after dinner. The program offered campus walks, strolls along the gorges, tours of the new library, and talks on the history of the campus buildings, and I took advantage of these. There were opportunities to exchange life stories with people you were not likely to see again, people with a wide variety of backgrounds and experiences. It was a chance for me to see where I fit into the world.

I enjoyed the week's session tremendously, and found that it had helped me grow. I could introduce myself to new people and talk about my situation with an ease that had come from simply doing it over and over. I met people from Barry's college class, and I was able to tell them about him. I could see the sympathy in their eyes; and I could say that yes, it was sad, but I was doing okay. By the end of the week, I felt a new confidence. When I hugged Barry's cousin good-bye, I drove home with a new attitude: I felt confident and sure of myself, and proud.

It was late July when I made my last trip of the summer. I drove Barry's Jeep across the country to Bozeman, Montana, to meet Sara and Richard, who were flying in from Alaska. A cousin of mine and her husband joined me for this adventure. We three are so different: I move fast; they are relaxed and laid-back. But we all wanted to make this trip together, so we gave each other the leeway to be ourselves, and it worked.

We retraced the route I had driven six years earlier with Barry before his illness, on our way to visit Sara and Richard in Seattle. As difficult as the trip was, now I relished it and I knew I was lucky to be able to do it with close family members. They both understood and supported me when I was overcome with emotion. But we laughed a lot, too. My cousin cannot get through the day without her afternoon ice cream, so we made sure to have our daily treat wherever we found ourselves each day as we crossed the country.

We sped through Pennsylvania, Ohio, Indiana, and Illinois, then north to Wisconsin, Minnesota, South Dakota, Wyoming, and, finally, to Montana. It felt strange to drive Barry's Jeep farther and farther from home, and even stranger when we stopped to browse the truck stops along the way, something Barry had enjoyed so much. He loved being on the road and the gritty atmosphere of truck stops.

My cousins turned out to be good companions. They had a great sense of humor, which had become my main criterion for friendship. We stopped in small towns along the way, and visited parks and museums, making it a vacation. We stayed overnight in La Crosse, Wisconsin, and walked beside the Mississippi River. In South Dakota, we visited a Native American tribal museum in the small town of Chamberlain. Further on, as we drove through the Badlands in a drizzling rain, the car became covered in mud that hardened to something like cement. It was pouring when we reached Mount Rushmore and the monument was half-hidden in mist and fog. We took a detour in Wyoming to visit Devil's Tower, hiked all around it, and lingered to watch the prairie dogs in their colonies. We even visited a Spam Museum somewhere along the way, something I protested, but my cousin thought it was just too funny to pass up. I gave in, and she photographed me in front of it, just to rub it in.

When we reached Bozeman, the Jeep was caked with mud. We spent an entire morning at a car wash, scrubbing and vacuuming. When we met Sara and Richard at the Bozeman airport, the car was spotless, and the young people were thrilled. Now it was their turn to get it dirty again when they drove it all the way back to their home in Fairbanks.

We stayed together for a few days at the home of some friends of my cousin, just outside of Bozeman. We took two days to drive through Yellowstone National Park. We marveled together at the boiling geysers and mud pots, and drove to various sites to search for wildlife. We were happy to be together, and yet conscious of Barry's absence. One day, when we were lost in the middle of Yellowstone, and unable to decide which direction to take at a crossroads, with each of us offering a different opinion, Richard said he could hear Barry chuckling at our predicament.

What a wonderful vacation it was, and how good to see Sara and her husband in this new setting, after all we had been through together. When we had to say good-bye, we put them on the road heading west, and my cousins took me to the airport to fly back east, while they continued on their own vacation. I felt Barry with me as I flew from Bozeman to our home in New York.

CHAPTER SIXTY-EIGHT

END OF SUMMER

As my first summer alone drew to a close, Dr. Lewis invited me to a beach party at his home in Connecticut. I wanted to go, but I was more than a little reluctant. I hadn't been to any parties by myself yet, and I wondered how it would feel. I didn't know how to act as a widow at a party. Still, I knew that it would be better to go than to stay at home, hiding from life. So I picked myself up, and found my way to another new experience.

I walked into Dr. Lewis's home and found myself in the midst of strangers celebrating life. Nobody asked me why I was there by myself. I didn't have to explain my circumstances to anyone. People had come to have a good time, to enjoy life and each other, and I did my best. I was grateful to be included in this party, and tried to take a lesson from this remarkable man, who had taught me to relish the life we have while we have it.

A month later, I attended another significant occasion: a dedication ceremony at our local hospital in Barry's honor. We had set up a memorial fund for Barry, and friends and family had been contributing to it all these months. Now a piece of much-needed equipment, a portable slit-lamp, had been purchased for the ophthalmology department at the hospital, and a beautiful plaque had been engraved in appreciation of Barry's work there.

The dedication was to take place at the end of a hospital staff meeting, and I was invited to attend. I walked into the group of my husband's colleagues and sat down in the back of the room. I had never been to a hospital staff meeting, though I had waited at home many evenings while Barry attended them. Invariably, he would come home vowing never to go again because the meeting had been so boring. I smiled to myself at the memory. Wouldn't he laugh to know that I was here, and wouldn't he be amazed at this fond dedication in his memory? He had told me so many times that once doctors retired from the hospital staff they seemed to be forgotten immediately. Not Barry.

Again I felt Barry's spirit with me here. Was it my imagination? I don't think so. Too many coincidences have occurred; there is too much to ignore. I feel someone near me; I sense Barry is telling me how to do something, something I wouldn't normally know how to do. Family members have heard him or felt him near. How to explain this? It is not understandable, and I just take as it comes, letting the experience unfold. I have come to believe that there is much we do not know and cannot know.

CHAPTER SIXTY-NINE

ENDING (FALL 2002)

It is time for me to end this chronicle. This journal started out as a way for me to record the details of Barry's illness as we were going through it. It was hard to remember all the facts and to keep them straight in my mind, so I started writing them down in an effort to clear my head. I found that as I wrote, I felt a release, and so I continued. At one point, Barry started reading this journal. He liked it.

I never dreamed that it would end this way. I was hopeful all the way through. I still think that that is a good way to be, and a good way to handle serious illness. I have learned this attitude from people working in the field. Barry and I met so many kind and compassionate people along the way, and we had some powerful experiences. I prefer to think that we had a wonderful and loving four years, rather than four difficult years. Both are true.

And forgiveness is finally coming to me. I forgive Barry and I forgive myself. This elusive feeling arrived after I finally stopped searching for it. Even though I realized that forgiveness would help me more than anyone, that forgiveness was really for ME, I still couldn't let go of my anger. I didn't feel that I could ever forgive either Barry or myself for our mistakes. I gave up trying. I finally accepted the fact that I couldn't do it. I surrendered. I told myself that this was okay and I would just move on and pay attention to the present and my future, and leave the past alone. It was only when I gave up the struggle that my resentment faded. I didn't need it any more. That brought me peace.

Although I do not know what lies ahead for me, this chapter is over. I wanted to document our four years' journey into illness and through it, to record what it feels like to deal with cancer; and to tell of the wonderful, generous souls who helped us cope. Our love grew stronger during these four challenging years, and I carry that with me always. Our relationship with our family deepened. Even in the depths of sadness, the end of Barry's life was a spiritual experience for all of us. Something miraculous was revealed to us: the strength and beauty of the human spirit. I am deeply thankful for that. I will never be the same.

THE END FOR NOW

****

POSTSCRIPT
THE YEAR 2003

It is now early in the year 2003. I have lived for more than a year without my husband. I want to write one last note in this journal. Every time I think I have reached the end of this saga, I sense that I am changing again, and I want to write about it.

This year we are having a real winter: a cold, snowy, icy winter. I have lost electrical power in the house several times, but I have handled it. I have shoveled the walk and my driveway has been plowed. I have driven on our hilly, twisty roads in my four-wheel-drive car in the middle of snowstorms. I am managing. Barely.

Something changes in a grieving spouse after the one-year mark. You have lived through the entire cycle; you have passed all the anniversaries once. You have made it through what you knew you couldn't. At the one-year date, I felt happy that I had lived through that period. I felt elated, in fact. I felt that I could make it, that I had made it, that I was a survivor. Of course my family was here with me, celebrating the holidays. Together we held a ceremony unveiling Barry's headstone. So I was not alone. I had the people here with me who had helped me through the period a year ago when my husband passed away. Lucky, again.

After the family left, I found myself quite alone. I began to feel unbearably sad. I still visited Barry's grave almost every day. When would I feel comfortable leaving this ritual behind? I was afraid of becoming a professional widow. The first year of grieving was over - shouldn't I feel better? The sad truth is that the hard, cold facts will not change: all I will ever have are memories. I will never feel my partner beside me again; I will never reach over in bed and touch him. I will never feel better, if by that I mean that I will not miss him too much, not yearn for just one more day or night together, not cry over how much we once had. So I had better get on with it. "Get on with it" -- what a phrase. How many well-meaning relatives have urged me to do that? They just want to see me "settled," dating, in a relationship, and not reminding them of such loneliness and sadness.

There is always the prospect of re-marrying or finding a new companion. Right now, that thought makes me cringe. I have visions of an attractive gray-haired man asking me out to dinner, but then I see myself bursting into tears. I remember Barry's words, a few days before he died, telling me to remarry; and just in case I wasn't paying attention, he told our daughters, too. He didn't want me to be alone. I bless him for that, for it may take away some of the guilt if that unlikely situation should ever arise. But now I know that I can live alone, and that there are worse things than being single. I met Barry when I was eighteen years old; how different it would be to meet someone at this age. Yet, I know that some people do, and find happiness. Perhaps - I will not rule it out.

Meanwhile I am building a life. I have two volunteer jobs, both meaningful, but one of which I really love. It is intense work, with people I enjoy, performing a difficult but worthwhile task. We find free flights for cancer patients on corporate jets with empty seats. Some of the patients are in crisis and we get the corporate flight schedules only a week in advance, so matching the two can be difficult. I go home from this job tired but happy, knowing that I have done something good that I am proud of. I have entered a new workplace, met new people, made friends, and presented myself as the person I am now. I am not half of anything any more; I am a "whole" myself.

I have developed a circle of friends, almost all women, who like to do the things I enjoy: walking, going to movies, visiting museums, eating out. Occasionally, I go out with couples, friends Barry and I used to enjoy spending time with. Sometimes we go to the city to see one of Ellen's plays. Sometimes I go out with swimming buddies or karate friends. People are kind to me, and I am grateful. I still faithfully swim every morning, and go to my karate classes two or three times a week. These activities have been life-savers for me, both because of the physical outlet, and because of the wonderful people there.

At last, I have been able to create art again. It has taken me all this time to be able to pick up my tools and work. I had worked on old projects, but had not been able to start anything new. Now, finally, I am working on a new piece. It is somewhat different from my old work, and very satisfying.

And I am planning more vacations for this year. At last, I will return to Arizona in the spring, a place I have sorely missed. I was there last with Barry in 2000, when our daughters surprised him by joining us. I think this will be the most difficult journey for me, but I know I have to do it. I am aching to do it. I will be joined by a friend who used to work in our office, so she knew Barry well. I will visit some of the beautiful places I love, and hope my husband's spirit will be with me. I think it will be. I am also planning a trip to Alaska this summer, with a friend and my cousin and her husband. We plan a short cruise and a week with Sara and Richard in Fairbanks - a real treat.

The challenge now is to recover meaning in my life. I used to have meaning - lots of it - I took care of my family, and then Barry's office, and then, finally, I joined him in his battle with cancer. That really was my life. It ended abruptly. Now it is as if my job is over. But I still feel young, and I don't want to just look back or sit around for the rest of my life. I am trying to find meaning in my volunteer work and in my family. I still want to make a contribution. I know I can do it, but the task is a lonely one. It is a struggle, but worthwhile things take effort. It will be well worth it.

This is where I am right now. Happy to be alive; enjoying every day I can; still crying over my loss. I know that what I make of the rest of my life is up to me. I feel this as I have never felt it before. I can do it at my own pace. And I will. I know I will. And when it is all over, I know now that it will not be the end.

****

About the Author

Nancy Greyson Beckerman is a mother, teacher, artist, swimmer, student of karate, docent, caregiver, and medical office manager.

In 1998 Beckerman's husband of 33 years was diagnosed with sarcoma, a deadly form of cancer. For the next four years, the couple fought the disease together, managing to take vacations and celebrate family occasions, in between cancer treatments.

Beckerman started keeping a journal during this time, and continued writing for about a year after her husband's passing. This manuscript is the result of that endeavor.

CPSIA information can be obtained at www.ICGtesting.com
Printed in the USA
BVOW040016061211

277672BV00001B/7/P